HEALTH & WEIGHT-LOSS
BREAKTHROUGHS 2010

HEALTH & WEIGHT-LOSS
BREAKTHROUGHS 2010

SELF-CARE SOLUTIONS TO FEEL & BE YOUR BEST

FROM THE EDITORS OF **Prevention**

RODALE

Photo credits are on page 356.

978-1-60529-711-8

2   4   6   8   10   9   7   5   3   1   hardcover

We inspire and enable people to improve their lives and the world around them

For more of our products visit **rodalestore.com** or call 800-848-4735

CONTENTS

PART 3
FITNESS MOVES

PART 4
NUTRITION NEWS

PART 5
MIND MATTERS

PART 6
BEAUTY BREAKTHROUGHS

INTRODUCTION

WE LIVE IN SUCH AN AMAZING TIME; new discoveries are made every day that can change our lives for the better. But if you don't know about them, they can't help! We've filled this book with all of the newest, most cutting-edge research and advice, to help you live better each day.

In Part 1: Health Breakthroughs, you'll discover the top medical advances, amazing innovations that can protect your heart, fight cancer, and improve how you feel. You'll learn about cures your doctor might not even know about. And you'll be pleased to know that you're doing so many things right, and you'll be surprised by the signs we've uncovered that show you'll live longer than you think. You'll also find out about simple changes to make your home healthier than ever.

Part 2: Weight-Loss Wisdom offers the latest research in weight loss. You'll discover how five frustrated women busted through plateaus and lost weight for good. See the simple food swaps that will help boost the benefits of your workout and burn more fat. You'll also learn how spirituality was the secret for some women to break their cycle of emotional eating and lose stubborn pounds.

Next you'll find our *Prevention*-exclusive, Weight-Loss Special Report: Tips, Tricks, and Techniques of the Stars of *The Biggest Loser*. They've lost weight, big time, and here they tell you how you can, too!

You'll be inspired to get moving by Part 3: Fitness Moves. You can lose up to 10 pounds—and look up to 10 years younger—with the Years-Off Workout. Sculpt your midsection even more next with our fastest-ever routine. Firm up flabby arms in just 10 minutes a day. And then look better from behind with our award-winning butt moves.

In Part 4: Nutrition News, you'll learn how to supercharge your menu—without supersizing your body. First, take our quiz to determine your nutrition IQ. Then learn strategies to make a good diet great: simple, smart ways to stock your pantry and refrigerator with healthy foods and make it easier to eat well. Even if your family loves the "white diet" (white pasta, white rice, white bread), you can get them to eat more greens—and reds and oranges—with our novel strategies.

You'll improve your mental well-being with the new strategies in Part 5: Mind Matters. Boost your brainpower so you'll remember more. Learn how to bust fatigue and energize your life. Discover how to prolong the best moments in life and strengthen all of your relationships.

In Part 6: Beauty Basics, you'll see how to look younger—without going broke. Learn new ways to keep stress off of your face and restore your smooth, even, youthful glow. Watch how five women updated their beauty regimens to achieve smoother, firmer, more radiant skin—and how you can, too. Finally, beautify three key age-betrayers: your neck, your hands, and your feet.

We hope this book helps you to truly feel—make that *be*—your best!

Part 1

HEALTH
Breakthroughs

CHAPTER 1

TOP MEDICAL
Breakthroughs

These amazing innovations in women's health can protect your heart, fight cancer, and improve how you feel every day

Enough medical studies are published each year to down a small forest. Most appear with little fanfare and fade quietly, of interest only to a small group of scientists. But last year a handful hit like small bombshells, overturning conventional wisdom about serious but common conditions. We culled the journals and queried the experts to find the biggest breakthroughs: the best new tests, drugs, gadgets, and procedures, and the new thinking about what we should do right now to stay healthy.

BREAKTHROUGH THAT CAN: SUPERCHARGE YOUR MENU (FOR NO EXTRA CALORIES)

Finally, an answer to the supermarket aisle question: Are organics worth the extra cost? A review of nearly 100 studies shows that the average levels of nearly a dozen nutrients are 25 percent higher in organic fruit, veggies, and grains than in conventionally grown produce. In some studies, organic options had nearly 50 percent more of the antioxidants quercetin and beta-carotene.

Stay healthy. Buy organic produce when you can. It's pricier, but you get more bang for your buck, says Kathleen Merrigan, PhD, assistant professor of nutrition at Tufts University. And that's not counting the benefits that come from reducing the amount of pesticides that enter the groundwater—and your body.

"You'll really do your health good if you splurge on organic as much as possible in the produce aisle," she says. If you have to be selective, she adds, pick organic versions of the fruits and vegetables that tend to have the highest pesticide residues. For a list of the most contaminated produce—plus other buying tips—go to prevention.com/budgetorganic.

BREAKTHROUGH THAT CAN:
MAKE YOU A HERO

If you witness someone collapsing, experts have long advised full-throttle CPR—chest compressions plus "rescue breaths." But recently, the American Heart Association announced a dramatic change: no more mouth-to-mouth for adults, because three studies have shown that chest compressions alone save just as many lives.

→ PREVENTION
Alert!

THE FOUR KEYS TO LONGEVITY

The following health habits can add years to your life. Talk about universal health insurance: If 90 percent of Americans got recommended mammograms, colonoscopies, and flu shots, 29,700 lives would be saved next year, according to the Partnership for Prevention. Fewer than half of adults over age 50 are up-to-date on colonoscopy screening, only 67 percent of women over 40 had a mammogram in the last 2 years, and a paltry 37 percent of adults get an annual flu shot. The fourth (and biggest) lifesaver: a daily low-dose aspirin, which would save 45,000 more lives.

Two-thirds of witnesses don't come to the aid of someone in need, often because they're worried they'll do CPR incorrectly, says Michael Sayre, MD, the lead author of the recent AHA advisory. "We hope this gets more people to act, because a victim who gets any kind of CPR more than doubles his chance of recovery," Dr. Sayre says.

Save a life. If you see an adult collapse, call 911, then use both hands to push hard and fast (to the beat of the Bee Gees' "Stayin' Alive"). Traditional CPR is best if you come upon an adult who's already unconscious, if the victim is a child, or in cases of drowning.

BREAKTHROUGH THAT: TREATS SINUS INFECTIONS THE RIGHT WAY

You know you should avoid antibiotics whenever possible to prevent the growth of drug-resistant bugs. Still, even doctors tend to think the drugs are necessary for sinus infections if symptoms last beyond a week or so.

But when researchers at Switzerland's Basel Institute for Clinical Epidemiology examined nine studies involving more than 2,500 adults, they found that the drugs almost never sped recovery. Even most of the people with a classic sign of severe infection—greenish mucus—improved just as fast by waiting as by taking meds. Antibiotics are powerless against viruses, the cause of most sinus infections, says allergist Neil L. Kao, MD, a member of the rhinitis/sinusitis committee of the American College of Allergy, Asthma & Immunology. The study shows that you shouldn't take antibiotics unless you have multiple symptoms, including facial pain, fever, pus, and more than a weeklong illness, he says.

Stay healthy. Don't bother going to the doctor unless you have multiple symptoms or the pain is unbearably intense, Dr. Kao advises. You'll get just as much relief with the following steps: Take a decongestant (avoid combo formulations with other active ingredients) and/or a mucus thinner. Rinse sinuses at least four times daily: Using a squeeze bottle containing $\frac{1}{2}$ teaspoon of salt in 8 ounces of tap water, bend your head down over a sink, squirt the solution into your nose, and let it run out. Take acetaminophen or another painkiller as needed for discomfort.

BREAKTHROUGH THAT CAN: HELP YOU CONTROL HUNGER AND LOSE WEIGHT

A kind of dietary fiber known as "resistant starch" is emerging as a new weight-loss powerhouse. A 2008 Swedish study found that people who ate a resistant starch at supper (in the form of barley bread) felt much less hungry than those who munched on plain white bread, and the hunger-quenching effect lasted past breakfast the next day.

Found in beans, slightly green bananas, and potatoes (white and sweet), among other foods, this kind of fiber "resists" being digested. Because the starch doesn't enter your bloodstream, it stabilizes blood sugar levels and may lower diabetes risk. It also boosts levels of healthful bacteria that nurture the immune system.

Stay healthy. Load up your diet with these indigestible carbohydrates, which are also found in brown rice and corn, says Leslie Bonci, RD, author of the *American Dietetic Association Guide to Better Digestion*.

Because the starch becomes resistant during cooling, serve these foods at room temperature or from the fridge: Think three-bean or (low-fat mayo) potato salad. You can find foods fortified with a resistant starch made from corn under the brand name Hi-maize. (Check out our picks at prevention. com/starch.)

"If you're eliminating carbs to watch your weight, you're not doing yourself any favors," Bonci says. "Adding these starches is an easy way to control both hunger and blood sugar."

BREAKTHROUGH THAT: IMPROVES OSTEOPOROSIS TREATMENT

A new risk calculator called FRAX helps you know if you really need bone-building drugs. Doctors have long disagreed about what to suggest for women with borderline results on a bone mineral density (BMD) test; some prescribe the drugs and some don't. The result, experts say, is that many women take the meds years before they really need to, facing side effects that range from stomach upset to esophageal ulcers.

PREVENTION
Alert!

THE BEST NEW HEALTH TOOLS

These drugs, tests, and devices are fresh on the market. Some are for use in the hospital, while others are meant for your medicine cabinet. Experts say all of them are a major boon to your health.

A DRUG THAT BRINGS FASTER HELP FOR MIGRAINES. Treximet, approved in 2008, combines sumatriptan (found in Imitrex) and naproxen sodium (Aleve), but it's 48 percent more effective than naproxen alone, and it has 28 percent more oomph than solo sumatriptan. The study, funded by drug maker GlaxoSmith-Kline, involved almost 3,000 migraine sufferers and was published in the *Journal of the American Medical Association*.

AN INJECTION THAT EASES A TRIP TO THE DENTIST. An innovative injected med called OraVerse reverses the effects of local anesthesia once your dental work is done, reducing the time you're numb by more than an hour.

A PATCH THAT TARGETS PAIN. The prescription Flector Patch, the first "skin delivery system" of an NSAID in the United States, puts only one-hundredth as much medicine into your bloodstream as a pain pill, studies show. Yet it relieves minor sprains and bruises just as well.

A BANDAGE THAT STOPS BLEEDING FASTER. Most bandages simply cover a wound, but the new BloodStop gauze actually stops the flow of blood in less than a minute. When hit by blood, BloodStop's materials turn into a gel that speeds coagulation. Nationally available in drugstores for the first time in 2008, it's especially useful for deep cuts or hard-to-stop nosebleeds and for people taking blood thinners.

A TEST THAT HELPS VANQUISH A DEADLY BUG. The new blood test BD GeneOhm StaphSR Assay tells your doctor within 2 hours whether you're infected with antibiotic-resistant staph, known as MRSA. Until now, a test took 2 days, which was long enough for the infection to spread to bones, joints, heart, and lungs.

But FRAX, developed by the World Health Organization, uses 12 factors that affect bone health (including your weight, family history of hip fracture, and certain drugs or illnesses) to determine your 10-year risk of breaking a bone. According to guidelines set by the National Osteoporosis Foundation, if a bone density test raises concerns about your skeletal strength, you shouldn't start on bone-boosting drugs unless FRAX puts your risk of a fracture above 20 percent over the next decade.

Stay healthy. Don't take bisphosphonates without checking your FRAX score. Get a BMD test at age 65, and ask your doctor to use the result in calculating your FRAX score. (If you've been on bone-sapping drugs such as long-term steroids or have other risk factors for osteoporosis, ask your doctor if you should be tested earlier.) Or crunch your numbers yourself, with or without a BMD score, at shef.ac.uk/frax.

BREAKTHROUGH THAT CAN: SAVE 47,000 LIVES A YEAR

Three major studies in 2008 gave long-sought guidance on the best way to treat diabetes, which kills an estimated 234,000 people yearly. The answer: You must hit the disease hard and early and use a number of approaches at

PREVENTION Alert!

NEVER HAVE A HEART ATTACK!

Here's some lifesaving advice: A huge study found that following these five lifestyle guidelines slashes heart attack risk by a whopping 92 percent. Incorporating just the first two into your routine cuts your risk by more than half.

Here's what researchers at Sweden's Karolinska Institutet and Boston University School of Medicine (who reviewed the histories of 24,444 women) say are the factors that count.

1. Moderate amount of alcohol: no more than half a glass of wine daily
2. Healthy diet: enjoy one based on fruits, vegetables, whole grains, fish, and legumes
3. Daily exercise: more than 40 minutes of daily walking plus 1 hour a week of more strenuous activity
4. Healthy body weight: waist size is 85 percent or less of your hip size (use a measuring tape)
5. Not smoking: never smoked, or stopped at least 1 year ago

once. In one of the studies, researchers didn't merely control glucose levels; they also used drugs to reduce high cholesterol, triglycerides, and blood pressure. The result: They slashed the risk of dying within 13 years by 20 percent.

In another trial, attempting to play catch-up by getting glucose under tight control in people with diabetes who were already older and sicker turned out to be so dangerous that the government stopped the study prematurely.

The third study showed that the body has something researchers call "metabolic memory": People who got their glucose levels way down right after diagnosis had a 13 percent lower risk of dying a full decade later—even if they'd let blood sugar ratchet up higher in the intervening years.

Stay healthy. The minute your doctor says your glucose levels aren't healthy, you must take action ASAP. "This is true even for people with prediabetes, because by the time the hammer of the full disease hits, a lot of damage is already done," says Stuart Weiss, MD, medical director of the Diabetes Education Center at New York University's Tisch Hospital. Get serious about eating healthy and exercising, and take the medications your doctor prescribes—including statins for cholesterol and drugs for high blood pressure.

BREAKTHROUGH THAT: KEEPS YOU OFF OF THE OPERATING TABLE

Arthroscopic surgery is no help at all for people with arthritic knees, concludes a recent study published in the *New England Journal of Medicine*. Nearly 200 adults with moderate-to-severe knee osteoarthritis had arthroscopy plus therapy, or physical and medical therapy alone—and 2 years later, the surgery group was no better off.

Arthroscopy remains an important tool when it comes to repairing cartilage tears and other injuries, says Robert Marx, MD, a knee and shoulder surgeon at the Hospital for Special Surgery in New York City. "But it's clear that you can't fix arthritis with arthroscopy," he says.

Stay healthy. Give your doctor a detailed account of your knee ache, including when it started and whether it came on gradually or suddenly. (Pain after a sharp twist is more likely to be caused by an injury.) You may need an x-ray, MRI

(continued on page 12)

Cutting-edge research reveals how music can help you ease pain, think smarter, feel energized, and fight disease.

Certified music therapists treat heart disease, asthma, Alzheimer's, and more. To find one near you, call the American Music Therapy Association at 301-589-3300. But you don't need to study music theory to reap the benefits. Here's how to find harmony between your physical and mental health.

In Pain? Try Music Plus Guided Imagery

Simply listening to music for 1 hour a day can ease your pain by 20 percent, Cleveland Clinic researchers recently found. It can even reduce the need for pain medication before and after surgery. Music seems to stimulate the release of pain-masking endorphins in the brain, says Cheryl Dileo, a music therapy professor and director of the Arts and Quality of Life Research Center at Temple University. Music can also amplify the effects of a visualization exercise called guided imagery, in which patients focus on a specific image or sensation that evokes the emotions they want to feel, says Ronit Azoulay, a music therapist at the Louis Armstrong Center for Music and Medicine at Beth Israel Medical Center in New York City.

SOUND ADVICE: To stage your own music-guided imagery session at home, find a comfy chair in a quiet place to sit with your eyes closed and feet up, suggests Joke Brandt, PhD, assistant director of the Arts and Quality of Life Research Center at Temple. If pain is limiting your mobility, select music that makes you feel energetic. If it's interfering with your sleep, choose tunes that make you feel relaxed.

Next, think of your favorite place or a calming image, such as a quiet stream or deserted beach, says Dr. Brandt. "Focus on your breathing and the sensations in your body. Imagine each of your senses reacting to this favorite place or image—the smells, the sounds, the sights. When these thoughts wander, focus on the music." Once the song stops, don't jump up. Sit and relax for another minute or two. Repeat daily.

Sleepless? Get in Tune with Your Brain Waves

People with insomnia who listened to classical piano created in response to their own brain waves—a technique called Brain Music Therapy—improved their sleep quality in 4 weeks, found a University of Toronto study. The cutting-edge therapy boosts levels of melatonin, which is a brain chemical linked to sleep.

SOUND ADVICE: For $550, you can get your own BMT CD to use at home. It's quick and easy: While you're in a relaxed state, doctors monitor and record your brain waves and then use a computer program to create unique, sleep-inducing piano passages using your own measurements. (Log on to brainmusictreatment.com for locations.) Listen to your 12-minute loop at bedtime with headphones to drift off into dreamland.

"Feeding your brain its own rhythms helps your muscles and breathing relax," says Galina Mindlin, MD, PhD, a supervising attending and assistant clinical professor of psychiatry at St. Luke's-Roosevelt Hospital Center in New York City.

Got the Blues? Listen to Upbeat Songs While You Walk

Listening to music can ease depression symptoms by up to 25 percent, Cleveland Clinic senior nurse-researcher Sandra Siedlecki, PhD, recently found. The benefits are physical, too. Focusing on New Age music reduced levels of the stress hormone cortisol, according to a recent French study, and research at the University of California, San Diego, revealed that listening to classical music lowered the blood pressure of college students.

A Japanese study concluded that your favorite workout tunes can ward off fatigue during exercise, which is another proven mood-lifter. This has convinced some experts that combining music and exercise is one of the best bulwarks against depression.

SOUND ADVICE: When trying to cheer up, resist the temptation to wallow in sad songs. Choose up-tempo tunes instead, Dileo suggests. Listening for just 10 to 20 minutes undisturbed can boost your mood.

Upbeat tunes can also energize you during a workout. Aim for at least 30 minutes of cardio, such as brisk walking, running, or biking, 5 days a week, because that amount can help reduce depression. Make sure the music and exercise rhythms are in sync. For a power workout, try the thunderous album *Sai-so: The Remix Project* by the Japanese drum group Kodo, recommends Nancy Buttenheim, director of Kripalu DansKinetics Teacher Training in Stockbridge, Massachusetts.

imaging, or both. If tests show arthritis, stick to physical therapy, pain-relieving medications, and, if needed, steroid injections. If your pain is severe and these treatments don't help, you might eventually need a knee replacement.

BREAKTHROUGH THAT CAN: HELP YOU KEEP YOUR BREASTS

A woman who has a lumpectomy for early-stage breast cancer faces a grueling 5 to 7 weeks of daily radiation treatment. That's a schedule so arduous for women with jobs or young children or who live miles from the clinic that they sometimes choose a mastectomy to avoid it.

Now results from a 12-year Canadian study have proven that a 3-week radiation regimen of slightly higher daily doses is just as effective—with no decrease in survival rates or breast appearance. That's convinced doctors, says Anthony Zietman, MD, radiation oncologist at Massachusetts General Hospital. For women who find the longer schedule overwhelming, this is a good option.

Stay healthy. Be vigilant about getting mammograms. This less-grueling treatment is appropriate only when cancer is detected early. If your doctor does recommend radiation, ask if you qualify for this shorter plan.

BREAKTHROUGH THAT MIGHT: PREVENT THOUSANDS OF CASES OF COLON CANCER

When doctors perform a colonoscopy, they typically look for polyps. But a study of 1,800 patients found that about 9 percent of those getting the exam had a different kind of growth—one that's flat or even recessed. Why that

93 PERCENTAGE OF COLON CANCER PATIENTS WHO SURVIVE 5+ YEARS WHEN THE DISEASE IS DETECTED EARLY, ACCORDING TO THE AMERICAN CANCER SOCIETY

EARLIER CANCER DETECTION

The following breakthroughs will someday dramatically change how doctors diagnose—and treat—cancer.

University of Texas doctors are developing a new lung cancer test via a simple mouth tissue sample. It compares genetic changes that take place 95 percent of the time in both mouth and lung cells.

Norwegian researchers are studying a new ultrasound device that can catch tiny tumors earlier, distinguishing different organs and injected contrast agents more clearly. It's now being evaluated in clinical trials.

Shining a new type of laser light on a patient's breath can detect precancerous cells, according to scientists from the National Institute of Standards and Technology and the University of Colorado at Boulder.

An Australian researcher has developed a noninvasive "virtual biopsy" technology using harmless electrical currents to better identify skin and cervical cancer and eliminate the need for diagnostic surgery.

In what's being hailed as a milestone in women's health, a team of researchers led by Yale University School of Medicine gynecologist Gil Mor, MD, PhD, has developed a simple blood test that was 99 percent accurate at detecting ovarian cancer in recent studies, even in the disease's earliest stages. The screening—which examines six proteins in a woman's blood—will become widely available after the results of its current phase III trial are approved as expected. Ovarian cancer kills more than 15,000 women a year; it's often symptomless and not found until advanced stages.

matters: These overlooked growths are up to 10 times as likely to be cancerous as equal-size polyps, the researchers found.

"These findings will make doctors more vigilant in searching for and removing these lesions, and that should slash the rate of colon cancer and even death," says gastroenterologist John L. Petrini, MD, president of the American Society for Gastrointestinal Endoscopy.

Stay healthy. Don't rush to get a "virtual" colonoscopy. Though another 2008 study found that an x-ray colon exam is almost as accurate as the old-fashioned kind at finding large polyps and cancers, experts don't think it's as good at detecting flat lesions—so it's safest to stick to a traditional colonoscopy for now, Dr. Petrini says. And when you have a colonoscopy scheduled, the new finding means it's more important than ever to follow the prep instructions: Only a clean colon will allow your doc to spot these less obvious growths.

BREAKTHROUGH THAT CAN: SLASH YOUR RISK OF DIABETES

Researchers have long believed that if your BMI is under 25 (meaning that you weigh less than 145 pounds if you're 5-foot-4, for instance), you're safe from the ill effects of obesity. But a recent study from the Mayo Clinic showed that many women are dangerously "skinny fat." More than half of the 1,101 women with a BMI under 25 actually had more than 30 percent body fat, making them "normal weight obese." Because fat cells pump out damaging hormones, these women had four times the rate of prediabetes of those with less body fat.

Stay healthy. You can't tell if you're skinny fat simply by looking in the mirror because excess fat cells can hide deep in your abdomen or distribute evenly over your arms and legs. So get your body fat percentage checked. A spa or health club is more likely than your doctor to have testing equipment.

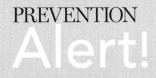

PREVENTION Alert!

HEAL FASTER WITH HYPNOSIS

Here's some mesmerizing news for breast cancer patients: Just 15 minutes of hypnotherapy can reduce the amount of anesthesia needed during surgery and the pain, nausea, and fatigue afterward. Doctors at New York City's Mount Sinai School of Medicine gave 200 women preoperative hypnosis or psychological consultation and also found the hypnosis patients were out of surgery 11 minutes earlier on average.

Find a licensed hypnotherapist at asch.net; hourly sessions usually cost between $100 and $150.

A device like the Bod Pod (which calculates how much air your body displaces when you sit in a closed booth) or a handheld or scalelike machine such as the Omron or Tanita brands (which measure the speed of an electrical signal zapping through your body) will do the trick, says study author Francisco Lopez-Jimenez, MD, a Mayo Clinic cardiologist. You can also buy one of the scales or handhelds for home use. They're not as accurate as a professional model but should be adequate for tracking your levels.

Over 30 percent fat? Don't just cut calories because then you'll lose lean tissue along with fat. Instead, add exercise. What's best: Combine cardio and strength training so you build muscle as you burn fat.

INNOVATIONS ON THE HORIZON

The following hot ideas could be available in the next couple of years.

Surgery that doesn't leave a scar: Using this approach, known as NOTES (for natural orifice translumenal endoscopic surgery), a surgeon makes not a single snip in your skin, working instead through openings such as the mouth or vagina. So far, the technique seems less painful and faster-healing, says NOTES pioneer Pankaj J. Pasricha, MD, at the Stanford University School of Medicine.

A drug that halves MS attacks: Current meds for the nerve-destroying disease multiple sclerosis prevent relapse in only 30 percent of patients. But with the new drug fingolimod, more than two-thirds of patients haven't had a single relapse in 3 years. A larger trial is in the works.

A test that's better at predicting women's heart risk: If you don't have obvious signs of heart problems, your doctor probably calculates your odds of developing cardiovascular disease in the next 10 years by using the Framingham risk score, which looks at your age and cholesterol, among other things. But that underestimates the danger for some women and overstates it for others.

Much better, according to an international review of studies, is adding a check of your "ankle brachial index," which compares your blood pressure in your arm to that at your ankle. Combining this with the Framingham score jumps about a third of us from low- to higher-risk levels, because blockages in leg arteries often mean similar jam-ups around your heart.

CHAPTER 2

CURES
YOUR DOCTOR
WON'T REVEAL

Your physician might be withholding vital treatment options out of personal bias, lack of training, or both. Here are life-changing options—many of them on the cutting edge— you should know about

Breast cancer survivor Janice Collins gave silicone implants the benefit of the doubt not once, but twice. The first surgery resulted in an infection, the second in a lopsided breast. Only a chance meeting with another breast cancer survivor led her to investigate the DIEP flap, a reconstruction that would use her own abdominal tissue to build a breast that feels and looks natural.

"Not even my own doctor had mentioned this procedure to me," says the

61-year-old probation administrator, who ultimately received a DIEP flap and couldn't be happier with it.

The technique is just one of several advantageous treatment options—for hip arthritis, uterine fibroids, depression, and other conditions—your doctor might not tell you about. The reasons are multiple: Your doctor might lack training in new, cutting-edge surgeries; it might be harder for him to obtain insurance coverage for a particular procedure; or he might simply be cautious about treatments that don't have decades of data backing them up. However, that doesn't mean you wouldn't want to be aware of all your choices—and have the chance to make the most educated decision about your health care. Here are four you should know more about.

HIP ARTHRITIS

The usual treatment: If you develop mild to moderate forms of osteoarthritis of the hip in your 40s, you're usually told to wait until you're 55 or 60 for a full or partial hip replacement, in which the entire neck and head of the thighbone (the femur) or just the head are replaced with metal parts. Though it may mean tolerating limited movement and chronic pain, there's a reason for waiting: Metal hips last up to 20 years, and in a recent British study, they lasted this long in only half of osteoarthritis patients under age 40.

Smart option: Hip resurfacing: In this procedure, surgeons reshape the top of the thighbone and cover it with a metal cap that sits inside a thin metal hip socket, blocking painful nerve endings on both sides. More bone is left intact than with a replacement, which makes any future surgeries or adjustments easier to perform and more likely to be successful.

Why it might be better: Instead of suffering for years until patients qualify for a hip replacement, they experience "a nearly complete end to pain," says William Macaulay, MD, director of the Center for Hip and Knee Replacement at New York–Presbyterian Hospital/Columbia. The FDA-approved Birmingham Hip System was still providing pain relief 5 years after surgery in 98 percent of patients during clinical trials. In foreign studies, 98 percent of resurfacing recipients in eight countries were satisfied 7 years later.

Why it's kept quiet: Hip resurfacing hasn't been available in the United States for very long. The procedure was approved by the FDA in 2006. And some doctors with many years of hip replacement experience are skeptical because it's so new, says James Rector, MD, an orthopedic surgeon in Boulder, Colorado. Additionally, there's not much long-term data on its efficacy yet— only 9 years' worth, to be exact. These factors explain why it makes up less than 4 percent of current US hip surgeries.

Real-life endorsement: By age 42, Charlie Post had arthritis in his left hip that made it impossible for him to sleep comfortably, and the Bantam, Connecticut, resident could no longer hit the ski slopes with his three teenage sons. Three different doctors told him he was too young for surgery.

"One said I'd have to be walking with a cane before I had a total hip replacement," Post says. A year later, he read about resurfacing on the Internet; less than a month after surgery, he was almost entirely pain free and able to sit comfortably in cars and planes again—even skiing with his sons by the end of that season. Though he might still need a replacement someday, "ultimately, it was worth it," he says.

HIP RESURFACING PROS

❐ It's available to middle-aged arthritis sufferers.

❐ It provides marked pain improvement in almost 98 percent of recipients 5 years later.

❐ Nearly all patients are satisfied.

HIP RESURFACING CONS

❐ Because the data goes back only 9 years, it's unclear how long resurfacing delays full hip replacement.

❐ Femur fractures occur in 1.5 percent of patients, though they're twice as likely in women.

❐ A doctor should check your bone density first.

UTERINE FIBROIDS

The usual treatment: For these painful noncancerous growths, many doctors suggest a hysterectomy—removing the uterus—as the "first line of defense," says Michael Broder, MD, president of the Partnership for Health Analytic Research in Los Angeles. In fact, about 60 percent of all hysterectomies are for uterine fibroids. The surgery virtually guarantees a cure, but it is not for women who want more children or fear psychological distress from such surgery.

Smart option: Uterine fibroid artery embolization (UAE): During this uterus-preserving procedure, a radiologist threads a catheter through the groin and into blood vessels going to the uterus. Tiny plugs block the blood supply, shriveling the fibroids.

Why it might be better: The womb-preserving procedure reduces heavy bleeding, pain, and pressure about 90 percent of the time, according to studies by UCLA and Thomas Jefferson University. Patients who get UAE have less pain on average a day after the procedure than those who undergo hysterectomy or myomectomy (a laparoscopic procedure), average a shorter stay in the hospital (4 days or less, compared with 6 for hysterectomy or myomectomy), and return to work quicker (about 20 days, versus 62 days after hysterectomy or myomectomy).

Why it's kept quiet: Turf wars between medical specialists and uneven insurance coverage are two big reasons, experts say.

"Gynecological surgeons feel they're giving their business away to radiologists if they suggest UAE over hysterectomy," says Francis Hutchins, MD, an adjunct professor of obstetrics and gynecology at Drexel University who has published studies on UAE.

The numbers illustrate the divide: In an unpublished pharmaceutical study of surgically treated fibroid sufferers, 83 percent had a hysterectomy, 15 percent had a myomectomy, and just 2 percent had UAE, according to Dr. Broder.

Real-life endorsement: Like most women over 40 hospitalized with severely bleeding fibroids, Kathy Moore was scheduled for a hysterectomy. But the Washington, DC–area resident found it unacceptable.

"The emotional trauma of that would have taken me years to get over," says Moore. Three years ago, she decided to try UAE. "The bloating, cramping, and heavy bleeding are now just a memory."

UAE PROS

❏ There's less pain initially and a faster recovery time, compared with hysterectomy and myomectomy.

❏ Symptoms improve 90 percent of the time.

UAE CONS

❏ It has a significant failure rate; 20 to 30 percent of women will need another UAE treatment or a hysterectomy.

❏ Patients miss an average of 3 weeks of work.

DEPRESSION

The usual treatment: Antidepressants, talk therapy, or a combo of both.

Smart option: Electroconvulsive shock therapy (ECT): Hollywood portrayals such as *One Flew Over the Cuckoo's Nest* and *Requiem for a Dream* haven't won "shock therapy" many fans, but it's not science fiction. Studies show ECT offers remarkable symptom relief. Today, outpatients are given general anesthesia and a muscle relaxant, so there are no dramatic muscle convulsions. The treatment lasts just a few seconds, and patients wake up a couple of minutes later. Scientists are still unclear how exactly it works (just as they are with more accepted antidepressant meds). ECT is administered 6 to 12 times over 1 month, depending on a patient's needs, according to the American Psychiatric Association.

Why it might be better. ECT boosted quality of life in nearly 80 percent of patients, Wake Forest University School of Medicine researchers found, and it relieved depression symptoms for 83 to 95 percent of patients in a North

Shore–Long Island Jewish Health System study, which was a greater success rate than the 50 to 70 percent who improve on antidepressant meds.

Why it's kept quiet: Though an estimated 19 million Americans are depressed in a given year, just 100,000 adults receive ECT annually, in part because of its past. Risks in the 1930s and 1940s were due to misuse of equipment, incorrect administration, and improperly trained staff. Today, given correctly, one of the main concerns is that ECT patients often develop varying degrees of memory impairment, says Charles Welch, MD, a psychiatrist at Massachusetts General Hospital in Boston. About 12 percent of patients suffer amnesia for as long as 6 months after treatment, especially if they're female. (Memory problems last just 4 to 8 weeks when electrodes are placed on only one side of the head.) Because of this and the associated costs—private insurers may approve only a few sessions at a time—APA guidelines state it's best for patients who haven't responded to meds or who prefer ECT to other treatments. Still, "There is an inappropriate reluctance on the part of psychiatrists to refer people to ECT," Dr. Welch says.

Real-life endorsement: Former Massachusetts First Lady Kitty Dukakis turned to ECT in 2001 after 17 years of depression that resisted other antidotes. She still undergoes a six-treatment series every 10 months. The memory

ECT PROS

❏ It has a success rate of 83 to 95 percent of patients going into remission.

❏ It improves the reported quality of life in nearly 80 percent of patients.

❏ It boosts the efficacy of antidepressants in some people.

ECT CONS

❏ Needs to be repeated every 6 to 12 months in most patients, to prevent relapses.

❏ Can cause partial memory loss, ranging from weeks to months.

❏ Requires anesthesia and muscle relaxants, raising costs.

loss she experiences—forgetting phone numbers and directions, mostly—are "a trade-off. I needed something much more dramatic than what antidepressants did for me," explains Dukakis, 71, who chronicled her experience in the 2006 book *Shock: The Healing Power of Electroconvulsive Therapy*. After the initial round of ECT, "I just felt that relief immediately," she says. "I remember waking up and seeing my husband and smiling—and I had not smiled for a long time. It has changed my life."

BREAST RECONSTRUCTION

The usual treatment: Federal law requires insurers to pay for breast reconstruction after a mastectomy—however you choose to do it. Yet the overwhelming majority of women are offered only saline or silicone implants.

Smart option: The DIEP flap: In this sophisticated operation, a plastic surgeon moves a patient's abdominal skin and fat to her chest, transferring and reattaching blood vessels and sometimes nerves in the process. Named for the deep inferior epigastric perforator abdominal blood vessels that are used, the DIEP flap is an advancement of the TRAM flap, which is a more common, slightly easier technique that sacrifices grafted abdominal muscles to build a new breast. The DIEP flap leaves these abdominal muscles intact; the surgeon pushes them aside briefly to remove tissue behind them.

Why it might be better: "Preserving the abdominal muscles means you can still lift your kids and do all your daily activities," says John Hijjawi, MD, an assistant professor of plastic surgery at the Medical College of Wisconsin. There's also a chance you can regain sensation in your breast. A study of 24 women at Methodist Hospital in Houston found that every woman who received a nerve transfer regained some sensation within 6 months. Patients have less post-op pain, a shorter recovery, and fewer abdominal hernias than those who get TRAM flaps, according to the University of Texas M. D. Anderson Cancer Center and Mayo Clinic studies, and a lower risk of the complications associated with implants (such as pain, asymmetry, and the need for future surgical replacement).

The DIEP flap's emotional benefits are also significant: "Many women don't think of it as a reconstruction. They think of it as a real breast," says Joshua L. Levine, MD, a plastic surgeon in New York.

Why it's kept quiet: Fewer than 100 surgeons in the country can do the surgery; thus, just 7 percent of US breast reconstructions in 2006 were DIEP flaps, says the American Society of Plastic Surgeons. And despite the Women's Health and Cancer Rights Act requiring insurers to cover postmastectomy reconstruction, surgeons and patients "may have to jump through hoops" to get coverage for the $30,000-plus DIEP flap surgery, admits Dr. Levine, delaying surgery for months or years.

Real-life endorsement: One Ohio breast cancer survivor fought for 18 months before her insurer approved DIEP flap coverage.

"All of us want to live, but you want a quality of life after cancer, and insurance companies are holding walls in front of women," says the 54-year-old woman, who requested anonymity because she's forbidden to discuss her insurance settlement. Despite the long wait, the cancer survivor says, "it is still the best thing I ever did."

DIEP FLAP PROS

❑ Looks and feels more natural than implants.

❑ There's the potential for sensation in the reconstructed breast.

❑ It's a built-in tummy tuck; reconstructed breasts gain fat and the belly loses it.

DIEP FLAP CONS

❑ The surgery lasts up to 12 hours, with an average of 4 days in the hospital.

❑ Cost: Might have to fight insurers to pay for it

HEALTH "RULES" YOU SHOULD BREAK

The food pyramid almost crushed Elaine Monarch. She'd always enjoyed whole wheat bread and the other healthy carbohydrates that form the pyramid's foundation, but her resolve to eat plenty of grains grew even stronger after she went to her doctor complaining of bloating and diarrhea. "He told me I needed more fiber in my diet," she says. "That advice practically killed me."

Monarch, it turns out, has celiac disease: Her immune system attacks the gluten from grains, damaging her small intestine in the process. The founder of the Celiac Disease Foundation, she is still diligent about consuming enough fiber, but these days she gets it from fruit, nuts, and supplements instead of grains.

Americans are constantly bombarded with expert health advice, and many of the messages are unquestionably right for everyone. No one will ever get sick from avoiding cigarettes or trans fats. But some of the most commonly repeated pieces of advice actually aren't meant for everyone. After all, the USDA couldn't equip its pyramid with a section just for people with celiac disease. Health recommendations are sometimes based on studies that didn't include a good cross section of the general public. And even when broadly representative studies trumpet a 94 percent success rate, that still leaves 6 people out of 100 looking for answers.

"What's good for the population as a whole is not necessarily good for a given individual," says Dan Roden, MD, assistant vice-chancellor for personalized medicine at Vanderbilt University.

So we took a look at some pieces of conventional wisdom that are truly wise—for most people. Then we asked the experts what you ought to do, just in case you're not completely average in every way. Feeling kind of special? This is for you.

Your Fitness Routine

SMART ADVICE: Vigorous workouts do more for you than moderate ones.

TAILOR IT IF YOU'RE SEDENTARY AND YOUR MAIN GOAL IS WEIGHT LOSS. If you work too hard—and tire too quickly—you may not burn enough calories to make a real dent in your weight.

(continued)

A 2003 study of 184 women found that walking at a moderate pace for at least 150 minutes each week for a year was just as slimming as working out more intensely for shorter periods of time. In fact, women assigned to long sessions of moderate exercise lost about the same amount as women who worked harder for shorter bursts—15 to 18 pounds, on average. To drop weight, exercise most days of the week at a pace that you can sustain for 30 to 40 minutes. You should be able to talk without gasping for air.

SMART ADVICE: Walking is the simplest way to get exercise; all you need are sneakers and a sidewalk.

TAILOR IT IF YOU HAVE HEART DISEASE AND IT'S A SMOGGY DAY. Studies show that the tiny particles in the air during a high-smog day can increase the risk of heart attack. Move your workout indoors on smoggy days (check airnow.gov for local air quality), and flick on the air conditioner. It can cut indoor pollutant levels by up to 50 percent.

SMART ADVICE: Every little bit of exercise gets you fitter—even housework.

TAILOR IT IF YOU'RE TRYING TO PREVENT OR TREAT HEART DISEASE. True, any activity is better than none, but sweeping or pulling weeds probably won't work your heart hard or long enough to significantly reduce the odds of clogged arteries, heart attack, or stroke.

Instead, do 30 minutes of moderately vigorous exercise four or five times a week to dramatically lower your heart risk. A study of nearly 40,000 women found that briskly walking at least 2 hours each week halved the risk of heart disease.

Your Food and Drink

SMART ADVICE: Eat plenty of leafy green vegetables.

TAILOR IT IF YOU TAKE THE BLOOD THINNER WARFARIN (COUMADIN). This drug prevents dangerous blood clots by blocking the action of vitamin K, which is needed to make clot-building compounds in the blood, but too much K in your diet can overwhelm your protection. The nutrient is especially abundant in dark green, leafy vegetables such as spinach, Swiss chard, and kale, so don't have more than one serving of any of these in a day.

SMART ADVICE: Drink at least 8 glasses of water every day.

TAILOR IT IF YOU HAVE BLADDER CONTROL PROBLEMS. You might be able to avoid leaks by cutting back a bit on fluids. Ask your doctor how much you should drink each day, and don't worry if it doesn't come close to the magical "eight-glass" rule. Nearly 20 percent of your water intake comes from food anyway, according to the National Health and Nutrition Examination Survey. If you're peeing at least every 8 hours and your urine is light colored, you're likely drinking enough.

Your Medications

SMART ADVICE: When it comes to blood pressure, lower is better.

TAILOR IT IF YOU HAVE CORONARY ARTERY DISEASE (CAD). Getting your blood pressure down—to about 120/80—can help you avoid a heart attack or stroke, but don't go much lower. You need a little extra pressure to push blood through your narrowed vessels. A study of more than 22,000 people with CAD found that cutting diastolic pressure (the bottom number) to less than 70 more than doubled the risk of a heart attack or death.

One exception: Low blood pressure didn't seem risky for CAD sufferers who'd had angioplasty to clear obstructed vessels or bypass surgery to reroute blood through a healthy new vessel.

SMART ADVICE: Acetaminophen is one of the safest pain relievers and a first-line choice for arthritis relief.

TAILOR IT IF YOU HAVE A GLASS OF WINE (OR ANY ALCOHOL) DAILY. There's already a warning on bottles of acetaminophen for people who have three or more drinks every day, noting that the combo can damage the liver. But even light drinking can prime the liver for trouble, says Donald Jensen, MD, a board member of the American Liver Foundation. Although 4 grams of acetaminophen is the recommended maximum daily dose, he says, you shouldn't exceed 2 grams of acetaminophen on any day you have even one drink.

CHAPTER 3

Your Medical Tests
EXPLAINED

*Here's what to expect before, during,
and after six common procedures*

After 40, we're more likely to need certain medical tests to preserve our health. Learning that you have to undergo something with a hard-to-pronounce name (what is a colposcopy, anyway?) can be unsettling, but it doesn't have to be. Here's what to expect during some of the most common procedures, and what doctors would demand for themselves if they were on the table.

COLONOSCOPY

You need it if: You turn 50, to check for growths in your colon (called polyps) that can become cancerous.

How it works: The day before your appointment (usually at a hospital or outpatient endoscopy center), you'll clean out your colon with the aid of liquid laxatives—what many people consider the most unpleasant part of the procedure.

The next day, after you're sedated through an IV, the gastroenterologist will ease a thin, flexible tube into your rectum that gently expands your colon with air. The doctor will pass the scope, which is fitted with a camera, through your entire colon, searching for and removing polyps. The procedure is painless. The examination takes 15 to 30 minutes; you can go home after a 45-minute recovery period.

Essential tips: Watermelon and sesame seeds can obscure the view of the bowel lining, so don't eat either for a few days beforehand. After the procedure, you'll be hungry, so have food ready to eat as soon as you get home.

You should get the results: Immediately. But if the doctor removed polyps, a test to check them for cancer can take a week.

COLPOSCOPY

You need it if: You've had an abnormal Pap test.

How it works: As in a regular pelvic exam, you lie on a table in your gynecologist's office with your feet in the stirrups and the walls of your vagina expanded with a speculum. Your doctor will use an instrument to keep your cervix open, which can pinch, and swab the area with a mild acid to clear mucus and make the cells easier to see. A colposcope is used to illuminate and

PREVENTION
Alert!

THE TEST YOU MIGHT NOT NEED

Colonoscopy ranks near the top of screenings people are eager to avoid—yet a new study at Virginia Commonwealth University Medical Center found that more than half of screened patients are urged to get a repeat test sooner than national guidelines call for.

The real rules: Average-risk patients (such as those with no family history) should be screened every 10 years starting at age 50, according to the US Preventive Services Task Force and the American Cancer Society. Those at higher risk should start earlier and test more often; the American Gastro-enterological Association suggests every 5 years from age 40.

If one or more polyps are found, patients may need to return every 3 to 6 years, says the AGA. Learn your risk factors and more at prevention.com/coloncancer.

SPLIT DECISION

Many people wonder if they could safely split a higher-dose pill for their prescribed dose. On one hand, this can save you up to 50 percent on drug costs, but there are caveats. The ideal candidate is a tablet that is scored (has a groove down the middle) on at least one side. Some of the tabs on the fit-to-split list below are unscored but are still deemed safe to cut. The pill to split should contain twice your prescribed dosage. Inexpensive pill splitters are widely available; slice only one tablet at a time, and take each half before cracking another because some pills degrade faster when opened. Meds to cut include the following:

FIT TO SPLIT:

Atorvastatin (Lipitor)

Citalopram (Celexa)

Clonazepam (Klonopin)

Finasteride (Proscar)

Lisinopril (Zestril)

Lovastatin (Mevacor)

Metformin (Glucophage)

Nefazodone (Serzone)

Olanzapine (Zyprexa)

Paroxetine (Paxil)

Pravastatin (Pravachol)

Quinapril (Accupril)

Rosuvastatin (Crestor)

Sertraline (Zoloft)

Sildenafil (Viagra)

Simvastatin (Zocor)

Tadalafil (Cialis)

Vardenafil (Levitra)

Note: This list is by no means complete! Check with your pharmacist and prescriber to see if your tablets are candidates for splitting.

DO NOT SPLIT:

Capsules or gel caps

Tablets that break into multiple pieces because you won't get an accurate dose

Sustained-release (SR) or extended-release (XR) tablets (A few such pills can be split; check with your prescriber.)

Enteric-coated tablets ("candylike" hard coating)

Tablets designed to be placed under the tongue (sublingual)

Tablets designed to be placed between the cheek and gum (buccal)

Certain two- or three-drug combination tablets (e.g., Capozide)

Narrow therapeutic index (NTI) drugs (e.g., warfarin, digoxin, lithium)

Note: There may be other reasons that tablets should not be split, so always check with your prescriber and pharmacist first.

magnify the area up to 60 times to examine cervical cells. If there are any abnormal spots, a small sample of the tissue is sent for testing.

Any soreness is minor after a biopsy, but don't have sex or use tampons for at least a week. Wear a sanitary pad, because spotting or a dark discharge is normal for a few days. You can usually resume everyday activities immediately.

Essential tips: Ask your doctor to apply some benzocaine gel to numb the area before the exam.

You should get the results: In 5 to 7 days.

ENDOMETRIAL ABLATION

You need it if: You're among the 20 percent of premenopausal women who have extremely heavy menstrual bleeding and medication has not worked.

How it works: Although this hospital (or outpatient surgery facility) procedure doesn't usually end periods, it can lighten them; many patients still have a menstrual cycle and experience some discharge and bleeding. After sedating you, the gynecological surgeon expands your uterus, usually by filling it with fluid. Next, a lighted viewing instrument and an electrical, laser, or thermal tool are inserted to burn away a thin layer of the uterine lining. You should be able to go home the same day. The procedure can irritate your bladder, causing you to pee more than usual. Minimal pain, some cramping, and a light, watery discharge are common for 1 to 3 weeks; take an NSAID painkiller and wear a sanitary pad. Don't use tampons, have sex, or exercise until your doctor says it's okay.

Essential tips: If you're perimenopausal or have never been pregnant, your cervix might be tight and you might need a cervix-softening medication.

You should get the results: It provides significant relief for 90 percent of women. If it works for you, you'll get the results within several months.

MOHS MICROGRAPHIC SURGERY

You need it if: You have skin cancer.

How it works: After numbing the lesion with local anesthetic, the surgeon removes the cancer one layer at a time to preserve the greatest amount of healthy skin and examines the tissue under a microscope. The surgeon keeps removing layers until there are no more cancerous cells. Small and shallow wounds heal without stitches; larger ones may need sutures or even skin grafts over several months. Excising each layer takes about 15 minutes; repairing the skin can take from 30 minutes to several hours. With local anesthetic, pain is minimal.

Afterward, expect some swelling or bruising, which can be lessened by icing, and moderate pain, eased with acetaminophen or an NSAID. For a day or two, some clear or pinkish-yellow liquid might drain from the site.

Essential tips: Avoid alcohol and aspirin, which can increase bleeding, for several days. Your surgery could take all day, with long waiting periods, so bring snacks, water, something to read and occupy time, and any meds you take during the day. Ask for dissolvable stitches so you don't have to return to have them removed.

You should get results: You'll leave the doctor's office cancer free. Scarring is minimal, even when grafts are needed.

STEREOTACTIC BREAST BIOPSY

You need it if: A mammogram or sonogram turns up a lump.

How it works: During the procedure, you lie facedown on an exam table, your breast protruding through an aperture. The radiologist compresses your breast in a mammogram-like machine and numbs it with local anesthetic. Then the doctor makes a tiny nick, inserts a needle, and vacuums out some tissue. Don't panic if you feel a lump at the site after the procedure. A little blood sometimes collects there, but it should go away in a few days to a few weeks. Don't exercise or lift anything heavy for a day or two.

Essential tips: If you have a cold, you might want to reschedule because the radiologist can't do the biopsy if you're coughing.

You should get the results: In 2 to 3 days.

STRESS ECHOCARDIOGRAM

You need it if: You've been experiencing chest pains or shortness of breath, or if you're older than 50, sedentary, and have diabetes, high blood pressure, or high cholesterol.

(continued on page 39)

RX FOR SAFETY

Viewers of the medical drama *House* have come to expect bizarre explanations for every symptom: A sudden case of the sweats might be the work of a 20-foot tapeworm. Or a hidden brain tumor. Or a 20-foot tapeworm with a hidden brain tumor.

If *House* mirrored real life, many episodes would center around a mundane culprit: a drug interaction. As Americans take more and more medications for everything from skittish stomachs to sluggish moods, clashes between drugs have fueled a new epidemic of unexpected, sometimes dangerous side effects and complications.

One recent study suggested that at least 1.3 million Americans have prescriptions for drugs that could cause problems if taken together, and that only counts people with health insurance. Although the overall toll is unknown, it's undoubtedly huge, experts say . . . and growing.

Of course, if you take many medications at the same time, or large doses of a few, you're more likely to run into a bad pairing, says Marietta Anthony, PhD, associate director of the Center for Education Research and Therapeutics at the University of Arizona. But even common items like drugstore pain relievers can clash with other meds. Scan our list: If you spot your prescription, be extra alert for signs of possible conflicts; then, talk to your doctor. And check our easy switches. You may be able to take a safer combo.

An SSRI for Depression

SUCH AS Selective serotonin reuptake inhibitors such as fluoxetine (Prozac), paroxetine (Paxil), or sertraline (Zoloft)

ONE POSSIBLE CONFLICT IS A triptan drug used to treat migraines, such as sumatriptan (Imitrex), naratriptan (Amerge), or zolmitriptan (Zomig)

HERE'S WHY: Triptans and this type of antidepressant both increase levels of the brain chemical serotonin. But too much serotonin can set off a chemical firestorm known as serotonin syndrome, causing mania, an increased heart rate, seizures, and even death. The syndrome is rare, but the threat is real, says John Horn, PharmD, a professor of pharmacy at the University of Washington and coauthor of The Top 100 Drug Interactions. In 2006, the FDA issued an advisory to the roughly 50,000 Americans who take both SSRIs and triptans. The advisory told users they didn't have to stop taking the drugs but cautioned them to be aware of the risk.

PROTECT YOURSELF: Most patients can continue taking both triptans and SSRIs as long as they watch for signs of serotonin syndrome, Horn says. If you notice troubling symptoms, stop taking the triptans and check with your doctor right away.

An SSRI for Depression

SUCH AS: Selective serotonin reuptake inhibitors such as fluoxetine (Prozac), paroxetine (Paxil), or sertraline (Zoloft)

ONE POSSIBLE CONFLICT IS: Chronic use of nonsteroidal anti-inflammatory drugs (NSAIDs), such as aspirin or ibuprofen.

HERE'S WHY: You may have heard that long-term use of NSAIDs can cause bleeding ulcers and other stomach troubles. What's less widely known is that adding an SSRI increases the risk. Serotonin is the culprit here, too. Normally, that hormone encourages blood platelets to stick together—but because platelets soak up less serotonin when you're on an SSRI, they may have trouble performing their number one job: clumping together to form clots and prevent excessive bleeding in the stomach and elsewhere.

PROTECT YOURSELF: Even if you take an SSRI, it's fine to pop a couple ibuprofen or aspirin for an occasional headache. But if you need several doses of a pain reliever each day—a common regimen for people with arthritis—take acetaminophen instead. It's not an NSAID, and it doesn't encourage bleeding.

Blood Pressure Medication

SUCH AS: Specifically ACE inhibitors, such as benazepril (Lotensin), or diuretics, such as furosemide (Lasix) or hydrochlorothiazide (HCTZ)

(continued)

ONE POSSIBLE CONFLICT: Chronic use of NSAIDs, such as aspirin or ibuprofen

HERE'S WHY: If you take daily NSAIDs, your painkillers could keep these kinds of blood pressure medications from doing their job. These drugs work by ridding the body of extra salt or water, or by shutting off production of a hormone that prompts blood vessels to narrow. If taken regularly, NSAIDs can block both of these actions—and the blood pressure benefit.

PROTECT YOURSELF: If you experience problems, you have two options (ask your doctor which is right for you). "You can switch to a different blood pressure medication," Horn says: BP drugs called calcium channel blockers (such as amlodipine, or Norvasc) aren't deterred by NSAIDs. Or swap the pain relievers—use acetaminophen instead.

A Quinolone Antibiotic

SUCH AS: Ciprofloxacin (Cipro), ofloxacin (Floxin), or levofloxacin (Levaquin) to treat a urinary tract infection, traveler's diarrhea, or other problem

ONE POSSIBLE CONFLIT: Over-the-counter antacids containing calcium, magnesium, or aluminum, like Tums, Rolaids, Maalox, or Mylanta

HERE'S WHY: Quinolone antibiotics have an unhealthy attraction to the metals in common antacids. Magnesium, aluminum, and (to a lesser extent) calcium quickly glom on to the germ killers, rendering them much less effective.

PROTECT YOURSELF: You don't have to put up with a sour stomach while you're battling an infection. Simply wait an hour or two after taking your antibiotic before reaching for the antacid.

A Common Cholesterol Drug

SUCH AS: Specifically lovastatin (Mevacor), simvastatin (Zocor), or atorvastatin (Lipitor);

ONE POSSIBLE CONFLICT IS: Macrolide antibiotics, such as clarithromycin (Biaxin) or Erythromycin; Azole antifungals taken orally, such as the prescription drugs ketoconazole (Nizoral) and itraconazole (Sporanox)

HERE'S WHY: Some antibiotics and antifungals can block enzymes that help break down these specific cholesterol drugs. As a result, you may end up with 4 to 10 times more cholesterol medication in your blood than your doctor intended—enough to greatly increase your risk of muscle or kidney damage.

PROTECT YOURSELF: You can simply take a break from Mevacor or Zocor if you need one of these specific antibiotics or antifungals, Horn says. (Once your infection clears up and you're off those drugs, you can safely go back to your cholesterol medication.) Or your doctor may be able to prescribe a different remedy for your infection.

A Corticosteroid for Asthma, Hay Fever, or Other Allergies

SUCH AS: Budesonide (Pulmicort, Rhinocort) or prednisone (Liquid Pred)

ONE POSSIBLE CONFLICT: Antibiotics, Antifungals, Antidepressants, A calcium channel blocker for blood pressure—specifically diltiazem (Cardizem) or verapamil hydrochloride (Calan)

HERE'S WHY: When you take a corticosteroid—whether in a pill or via inhaler—you depend on certain enzymes in your body to break the drug down after it's done the job. But recent studies suggest that a number of other medicines can block the action of these enzymes, potentially leading to a corticosteroid overdose, Horn says. That can cause Cushing's syndrome, in which you can gain weight in your upper body and develop hypertension, bruising, weakness, depression, acne, and excess hair growth.

PROTECT YOURSELF: The risk is greater if you're taking the corticosteroid in pill form (inhalers deliver a lower dose) or if you add a pill to your inhaler regimen, as people sometimes do for an allergy flare-up. Ask your doctor if any of your other medications could potentially slow the breakdown of the drug. Cushing's syndrome is reversible, but you don't want to suffer any longer than necessary. One safety valve: It takes time for corticosteroids to build up to toxic levels, so a short course of an antibiotic or antifungal shouldn't cause trouble.

(continued)

An Over-the-Counter Stimulant Laxative

SUCH AS: Such as Senokot or Dulcolax

ONE POSSIBLE CONFLICT: Blood pressure medications; Antiseizure drugs, such as phenytoin (Dilantin); Antibiotics; The blood thinner warfarin (Coumadin); The heart medicine digoxin (Lanoxin)

HERE'S WHY: Many medications need plenty of time to be properly absorbed, but stimulant laxatives can rush them through your system. The result: You may not get the benefit of a crucial prescription.

PROTECT YOURSELF: Talk with your doctor before adding a stimulant laxative to your routine. Generally, you can stay on the safe side by taking it at least 2 hours before or after any other medications.

The Blood Thinner Warfarin (Coumadin)

ONE POSSIBLE CONFLICT: NSAIDs (including aspirin and ibuprofen); Antibiotics—specifically metronidazole (Flagyl), trimethoprim/sulfamethoxazole (Bactrim), or quinolone antibiotics such as ciprofloxacin (Cipro); Antiseizure drugs

HERE'S WHY: Some of these meds multiply the effects of warfarin, greatly increasing the risk of uncontrolled internal bleeding. The reason: NSAIDs keep platelets from sticking together, which—like warfarin—interferes with the clotting of blood. And certain antibiotics slow the enzyme that breaks down warfarin, also raising the risk of increased bleeding. On the other hand, antiseizure drugs can speed the breakdown of warfarin: Your blood can get too thick, causing a dangerous clot.

PROTECT YOURSELF: Interactions involving warfarin are relatively common and can be very serious. If you're on warfarin, don't take any other medication unless your doctor says it's okay.

How it works: In her office, your cardiologist first screens your heart with an ultrasound machine to measure how well it works at rest. If you check out okay, you hop on a treadmill with the doctor standing beside you; electrodes attached to you monitor your heart rate on an electrocardiogram machine (EKG) and a cuff measures your blood pressure.

The treadmill starts off slowly and speeds up every few minutes until you are tired or the doctor stops the test because you have symptoms or an abnormal electrocardiogram. A technician screens your heart by ultrasound again, and the doctor monitors your blood pressure and heart rate to see how long they take to return to normal.

Essential tips: Don't apply body lotion beforehand or else the electrodes will slide off. Wear comfortable clothes and don't forget your sneakers. Avoid big meals and caffeine before your appointment. Note: You can't wear a bra during the test, so expect to bounce around a little.

You should get the results: Immediately for the blood pressure and EKG.

SOOTHE THE WAITING-FOR-RESULTS JITTERS

Try these natural anxiety relievers recommended by Shelley Wroth, MD, director of clinical services at the Duke Center for Integrative Medicine.

Studies show that listening to music you love will help keep you calm both before and during a procedure.

Concentrating on your breath elicits a relaxation response. Sprinkle a piece of cloth with lavender oil and use it during the breathing exercise.

Much research has proven acupuncture effective for post-op pain and nausea. For best results, start 3 to 4 weeks before your procedure and continue with a few sessions afterward when cleared by your physician.

Anxiously awaiting medical results? Journaling about your experience for 20 minutes can calm you and help you better process the experience.

CHAPTER 4

Surprising Signs You'll
LIVE LONGER

Cutting-edge research reveals what you're doing right, and then we tell you how to do it better

Consider this: In the 20th century, the average life expectancy shot up 30 years—the greatest gain in 5,000 years of human history. And this: Centenarians—folks who make it into the triple digits—aren't such an exclusive club anymore, increasing 51 percent from 1990 to 2000. How to account for these dramatic leaps? Advances in health, education, and disease prevention and treatments are high on the list—and that makes sense.

WHAT YOU'RE DOING RIGHT

What you might not know is that seemingly unimportant everyday habits, or circumstances in your past, can influence how long and how well you'll live. Here's the latest research on longevity—science-based signs you're on a long-life path, plus tips on how to get on track.

Sign: Your Mom Had You Young

If she was under age 25, you're twice as likely to live to 100 as someone born to an older mom, according to University of Chicago scientists. They suspect that younger moms' best eggs go first to fertilization, thus healthier offspring.

Sign: You're a Tea Lover

Both green and black teas contain a concentrated dose of catechins, which are substances that help blood vessels relax and protect your heart. In a study of more than 40,500 Japanese men and women, those who drank 5 or more cups of green tea every day had the lowest risk of dying from heart disease and stroke. Other studies involving black tea showed similar results.

You really need only 1 or 2 cups of tea daily to start doing your heart some good, but just make sure it's a fresh brew. Ready-to-drink teas (the kind you find in the supermarket beverage section) don't offer the same health benefits.

"Once water is added to tea leaves, their catechins degrade within a few days," says Jeffrey Blumberg, PhD, a professor of nutrition science and policy at Tufts University.

Also, some studies show that adding milk might eliminate tea's protective effects on the cardiovascular system, so stick to just lemon or honey.

Sign: You'd Rather Walk

"Fit" people—defined as those who walk for about 30 minutes a day—are more likely to live longer than those who walk less, regardless of how much body fat they have, according to a recent study of 2,603 men and women.

Similarly, overweight women can improve their heart health by adding just 10 minutes of activity to their daily routine, says recent research. So take a walk on your lunch hour, or do laps around the field while your kid is at soccer practice. Find ways to move a little more, every day.

Sign: You Skip Soda (Even Diet)

Scientists in Boston found that drinking one or more regular or diet colas every day doubles your risk of metabolic syndrome, which is a cluster of conditions, including high blood pressure, elevated insulin levels, and excess fat around the waist, that increase your chance of heart disease and diabetes.

One culprit could be the additive that gives soda its caramel color, which upped the risk of metabolic syndrome in animal studies. Scientists also speculate that soda drinkers regularly expose their tastebuds to natural or artificial sweeteners, conditioning themselves to prefer and crave sweeter foods, which may lead to weight gain, says Vasan S. Ramachandran, MD, a professor of medicine at Boston University School of Medicine and the study's lead researcher.

Better choices: Switch to tea if you need a caffeine hit. If it's fizz you're after, try sparkling water with a splash of juice. By controlling blood pressure and cholesterol levels, preventing diabetes, and not smoking, you can add 6 to $9\frac{1}{2}$ healthy years to your life.

Sign: You Have Strong Legs

Lower-body strength translates into good balance, flexibility, and endurance. As you get older, those attributes are key to reducing your risk of falls and injuries—particularly hip fractures, which often quickly lead to declining health. Up to 20 percent of hip-fracture patients die within 1 year because of complications from the trauma.

"Having weak thigh muscles is the number one predictor of frailty in old age," says Robert Butler, MD, president of the International Longevity Center–USA in New York City.

To strengthen them, target your quads with the "phantom chair" move, says Joan Price, author of *The Anytime, Anywhere Exercise Book*. Here's how: Stand with your back against a wall. Slowly walk your feet out and slide back down until you're in a seated position, ensuring your knees aren't beyond your toes and your lower back is pressed against the wall. Hold until your thighs tell you, Enough! Do this daily, increasing your hold by a few seconds each time.

Sign: You Eat Purple Food

Concord grapes, blueberries, red wine: They all get that deep, rich color from polyphenols, which are compounds that reduce heart disease risk and may also protect against Alzheimer's disease, according to new research. Polyphenols help keep blood vessels and arteries flexible and healthy.

"What's good for your coronary arteries is also good for your brain's blood vessels," says Robert Krikorian, PhD, director of the Cognitive Disorders Center at the University of Cincinnati. Preliminary animal studies suggest that adding dark grapes to your diet may improve brain function.

What's more, in a recent human study, researchers found that eating 1 or more cups of blueberries every day may improve communication between brain cells, enhancing your memory.

Sign: You Were a Healthy-Weight Teen

A study in the *Journal of Pediatrics* that followed 137 African Americans from birth to age 28 found that being overweight at age 14 increases your risk of developing type 2 diabetes in adulthood. Adults with diabetes are two to four times more likely to develop heart disease than those without the condition, according to the American Heart Association.

Sign: You Don't Like Burgers

A few palm-size servings (about $2\frac{1}{2}$ ounces) of beef, pork, or lamb now and then is no big deal, but eating more than 18 ounces of red meat per week ups your risk of colorectal cancer, which is the third most common type, according to a major report by the American Institute for Cancer Research. Colorectal cancer risk also rises by 42 percent with every $3\frac{1}{2}$-ounce serving of processed meat (such as hot dogs, bacon, and deli meats) eaten per day, the report determined.

Experts aren't sure why red and processed meats are so harmful, but one of their suspects is the carcinogens that can form when meat is grilled, smoked, or cured—or when preservatives, such as nitrates, are added.

"You can have an occasional hot dog at a baseball game, but just don't make it a habit," says Karen Collins, RD, a nutrition advisor at AICR. And when you do grill red meat, marinate it first, keep pieces small (kebab-size), and flip them often—all of which can help prevent carcinogens from forming. If you're baking or roasting it, keep the oven temp under 400°F.

Sign: You've Been a College Freshman

A recent Harvard Medical School study found that people with more than 12 years of formal education (even if it's only 1 year of college) live 18 months longer than those with fewer years of schooling. Why? The more education you have, the less likely you are to smoke. In fact, only about 10 percent of adults with an undergraduate degree smoke, compared with 35 percent of those with a high school education or less, according to the CDC.

Sign: You Really Like Your Friends

"Good interpersonal relationships act as a buffer against stress," says Micah Sadigh, PhD, an associate professor of psychology at Cedar Crest College. Knowing you have people who support you keeps you healthy, mentally and physically. Chronic stress weakens the immune system and ages cells faster, ultimately shortening life span by 4 to 8 years, according to one study. Not just any person will do, however. "You need friends you can talk to without being judged or criticized," says Dr. Sadigh.

Sign: Your Friends Are Healthy

If your closest friends gain weight, your chance of doing the same could increase by 57 percent, according to a study published in the *New England Journal of Medicine*.

"To maintain a healthy lifestyle, it's important to associate with people who have similar goals," says Nicholas A. Christakis, MD, PhD, the study's lead researcher. Join a weight-loss group, train with a pal for a charity walk, or meet friends at a park or mall.

Sign: You Embrace the Challenge

People who consider themselves self-disciplined, organized achievers live longer and have up to an 89 percent lower risk of developing Alzheimer's than the less conscientious, according to two studies. When you're good at focusing your attention, you use more brainpower, says the lead researcher in both studies, Robert S. Wilson, PhD, a professor of neurological sciences and psychology at Rush University Medical Center in Chicago.

Set personal or career goals, and challenge yourself to meet them by a certain time. Also, try new things to stimulate your brain. If you always read fiction, for example, pick up an autobiography instead. The next day, try to recall three facts you learned from the reading.

Sign: You Don't Have a Housekeeper

Just by vacuuming, mopping floors, or washing windows for a little more than an hour, the average person can burn about 285 calories, lowering risk of death by 30 percent, according to a study of 302 adults in their 70s and 80s.

Sign: You're a Flourisher

About 17 percent of Americans are flourishers, says a study in *American Psychologist*. They have a positive outlook on life, a sense of purpose and community, and are healthier than "languishers"—about 10 percent of adults who don't feel good about themselves. Most of us fall somewhere in between.

"We should strive to flourish, to find meaning in our lives," says Corey Keyes, PhD, a professor of sociology at Emory University. "In Sardinia and Okinawa, where people live the longest, hard work is important, but not more so than spending time with family, nurturing spirituality, and doing for others."

HOW TO DO IT BETTER

Now that you know what you're doing right, wouldn't it be great to do more, even better? It's easier than you think. You could cut your risk of heart disease, get fitter, and slow aging—not to mention protect your smile—in less time than it takes to watch a couple of commercials. Better health does take time, but not as much as you may think. Yes, you should exercise 30 minutes a day and sleep 7 to 8 hours a night. But top experts in nutrition, cardiovascular health, and cancer prevention know the supersimple, amazingly fast steps you can take to dramatically improve your well-being. So take a minute or so and boost your health in almost no time flat.

Fight Cancer

Eat the peel. The bulk of an apple's benefit lies in its skin. In a recent lab experiment, more than a dozen chemicals in the peels of Red Delicious apples inhibited the growth of breast, liver, and colon cancer cells. Investigator Rui Hai Liu, MD, PhD, an associate professor of food science at Cornell University, suspects that the peels of other apple varieties are also extra potent. Buy organic if you're concerned about exposure to pesticides.

Take the right supplements. Getting enough vitamin D and calcium brings a remarkable reduction in cancer risk, found a recent 4-year study at Creighton University. Women who took the combo reduced their overall risk by up to 77 percent.

"Vitamin D enhances your body's immune response, which is the first line of defense against cancer," says lead researcher Joan Lappe, PhD, RN, a professor of nursing and medicine. Your skin makes D when it's exposed to sunlight, but researchers say the best way to guarantee you get enough is with a pill. The 1,100 IU used in the Creighton study will do the trick (and is safe).

Slow Aging

Sniff some lavender or rosemary. The scent of lavender can bring you a restful night's sleep, but the plant can do you a world of good in daylight, too. In a recent study, volunteers sniffed the essential oils of lavender or rosemary for 5 minutes. Result: Levels of the stress hormone cortisol in saliva dropped as much as 24 percent. That's good, because the hormone increases blood pressure and suppresses the immune system. What's more, people who smelled low concentrations of lavender or high concentrations of rosemary were better at getting rid of free radicals, the pesky molecules believed to speed aging and disease.

Cut Cholesterol

Sprinkle pistachios on your salad. Researchers at Pennsylvania State University recently gave volunteers a pleasant task: Eat 1½ ounces (about a handful) of pistachios every day. At the end of 4 weeks, those who munched the nuts reduced their total cholesterol by an average of 6.7 percent and their LDL ("bad") cholesterol by 11.6 percent. That reduction has a major payoff: Cutting your total cholesterol by about 7 percent reduces your heart disease risk by 14 percent.

Pistachios are one of the best sources of plant sterols, compounds we know reduce absorption of cholesterol, says researcher Penny Kris-Etherton, PhD, RD, who led the study. Just remember, 1 ounce contains about 160 calories. So pour a little less dressing on your salad as you add some pistachios, or go easy on butter or oil on your veggies when you sprinkle them on top.

Replace sugar with buckwheat honey. This sweet substance has been used for medicinal purposes since ancient times; when it's applied to a wound, honey is a natural antibacterial salve.

Now researchers say that its benefits may be much more than skin deep. Test-tube studies show that honey slows the oxidation of LDL cholesterol; it's when LDL is oxidized that it can be laid down as plaque in blood vessels. The variety of honey best at slowing oxidation: buckwheat.

Cool Hot Flashes

Breathe deeply. Slow, deep abdominal breathing can reduce the frequency of hot flashes by about half, according to three recent studies. Estrogen withdrawal is partly to blame for hot flashes, but researchers believe that stress also plays a role by firing up the sympathetic nervous system, which is the part of your wiring responsible for the fight-or-flight response.

The fix: Breathe deeply to enlist the parasympathetic nervous system, which activates your body's relaxation response. That will slow heart rate, relax muscles, and lower blood pressure. Sit in a comfortable chair and allow your breath to deepen. Inhale through your nose; exhale through your mouth. Close your eyes to cut out distractions. Let your belly be soft. You want it to rise and fall with each breath.

Keep Your Vision Sharp

Eat an egg. No offense meant to carrots, but research shows eggs are an even better source of the eye-friendly antioxidants known as carotenoids. Lutein and zeaxanthin are the crucial carotenoids for vision—the only ones that benefit the retina's fragile macula, which is responsible for central vision.

Eggs don't contain as much lutein and zeaxanthin as dark green, leafy veggies, but your body is better able to absorb the antioxidants in eggs, says nutritional biochemist Elizabeth Johnson, PhD, at Tufts University.

Worried about cholesterol? Don't be: Eating an egg a day increases blood levels of lutein (by 26 percent) and zeaxanthin (by 38 percent) without raising cholesterol or triglyceride levels.

Reduce Dangerous Inflammation

Pour a bowl of whole grain cereal. Whole grains are about much more than "regularity"; they can save your life. The Iowa Women's Health Study, which has followed nearly 42,000 postmenopausal women for 15 years, reports that women who ate 11 or more servings of whole grains each week were about a third less likely to die of an inflammatory disorder than those who consumed the least. (What is an inflammatory disorder? Any condition marked by chronic inflammation, including diabetes, asthma, and heart disease.) Good choices include oatmeal, brown rice, dark bread, whole grain breakfast cereal, bulgur, and (hurray!) popcorn.

"Whole grains contain the biologically active parts of the plant," says study leader David R. Jacobs Jr., PhD, a professor of epidemiology and community health at the University of Minnesota. "What keeps the plant alive keeps the eater alive."

Build Muscle Strength

Stretch your legs. If you have tight leg muscles, you'll not only improve flexibility by stretching but also build strength, says a new study published in the *Clinical Journal of Sports Medicine.* For 6 weeks, 30 adults with tight hamstrings did a series of stretches 5 days a week. Investigators measured their flexibility and thigh-muscle strength at the start and end of the study. All that stretching loosened up tight muscles and increased their range of motion, but the hamstrings and the quads (the muscles at the back and front of the thighs) also became significantly stronger.

Boost Antioxidants

Add avocado to your salad. Vegetables have an unexpected downside: Many of them are virtually fat free, and you need fat in the meal to absorb cancer-fighting carotenoids. In recent Ohio State University research, volunteers were given a salad with and without a sliced avocado. Blood tests showed that those who ate the avocado got 5 times as much lutein, 7 times as much alpha-carotene, and a whopping 15 times as much beta-carotene as those who ate the salad without it.

Snack on dried figs. Dried fruits are known to be rich in antioxidants, but some of the less popular types are the most nutritious. Figs and dried plums (aka prunes) had the best overall nutrient scores, shows recent research at the University of Scranton. A handful of dried figs (about 1½ ounces) increased "antioxidant capacity"—the ability to neutralize free radicals—by 9 percent. That's more than double the increase seen after a cup of green tea.

Eat a fruit salad. Antioxidants love company: A mixture of oranges, apples, grapes, and blueberries provides five times the antioxidant power you get from eating the same fruits solo, says recent research by Dr. Liu, at Cornell.

Ingredients to toss into fruit salad, ranked in order of phenolic content (a type of plant chemical that cuts the risk of chronic disease): cranberries, apples, red grapes, strawberries, pineapples, bananas, peaches, oranges, and pears.

Keep Your Smile Healthy

Kiss your partner passionately. You enjoy a kiss for other reasons, but according to Anne Murray, DDS, a spokesperson for the Academy of General Dentistry, it increases saliva in your mouth, which cleans your teeth of the bacteria that can cause cavities. If, alas, you have no one to kiss, try sugar-free gum containing xylitol.

Protect Your Stomach from Bugs

Turn down your fridge. If the setting is over 40°F, your food is sitting in the danger zone—the temperature at which bacteria begin to multiply. Each year in the United States, more than 75 million people get sick from contaminated food and 5,000 die. So use an appliance thermometer to be sure the temp is low enough.

Prevent Headaches

Keep your head up. "Posture is one of the least understood and appreciated factors in head pain," says Roger Cady, MD, vice president of the National Headache Foundation. One of the leading posture pitfalls: forward head posture (FHP). When your neck juts forward, you have to tilt your head up to see, Dr. Cady explains, and that can compress the nerves and muscles at the base of the skull.

A common cause of FHP: slumping in front of a computer. Physical therapist Colleen Baker, who practices at the Headache Care Center in Springfield, Missouri, offers the following tricks to help you get your head on straight.

- Imagine a cord attached to the top of your head, pulling toward the ceiling.

- Periodically check to make sure your ear is in line with your shoulder.

- Set your computer to remind you every half hour to repeat the first two tips.

Stay Mentally Sharp

Have 2 cups of green tea daily. Studies have shown that green tea helps keep cholesterol in check and may lower cancer risk. Now researchers say the drink may also work to maintain cognitive function. A Japanese study of 1,000 people over age 70 found that those who drank 2 cups of green tea daily did better on a variety of tests of mental abilities (including memory), and the more green tea they drank, the better they performed.

It's possible that something else is responsible for the mental clarity, such as the socializing the Japanese tend to do over a cup. But the results might partially explain why rates of dementia, including Alzheimer's disease, are lower in Japan (where green tea is commonly consumed) than in the United States.

CHAPTER 5

Healthy Home
MAKEOVERS

*We reveal the surprising health dangers
in your home's hidden spaces, plus expert
advice on what to keep and what to toss, and
tips on how to store things to maximize
your health*

Your cabinets and closets are always there for you, faithfully storing whatever you cram into them. But "out of sight, out of mind" can end up meaning "out of date," and that's just one of the unhealthy situations that could be developing behind those closed doors. Mold may be growing. Poisons may be lurking. Accidents may be waiting to happen.

So follow our expert-approved cabinet-by-cabinet, closet-by-closet guide on which household items to keep, toss, or even add to your shopping list. Here's how to give your storage centers a makeover—and protect your family's health in the process.

UNDER THE KITCHEN SINK

Mold spores are everywhere, scouting for a damp place to settle down and raise a big family. Don't let them. Mold irritates eyes and airways, contributing to chronic sinus infections and asthma. So keep your cabinet dry. Then, stock it right.

Keep

All-purpose cleaners: Pick ones with an EPA Design for the Environment label, which indicates that the ingredients are as safe as possible for the environment and you. (For a list, go to prevention.com/links.) Or go natural: Mix equal parts white vinegar and water in a spray bottle to clean glass, says Anne Steinemann, PhD, professor of civil and environmental engineering and public affairs at the University of Washington. For wood floors, add 1 teaspoon each vegetable oil and vinegar to 1 quart of water. Mop with the solution, and then rinse with fresh water.

Rubber gloves. They protect your hands from hot water and cleaners that can irritate or dry out your skin. Choose ones that reach at least halfway up your forearm.

Dishrags: Longer-lasting than sponges, they are an environmentally friendly option for washing dishes and wiping counters. But bacteria can grow on dishrags, too, so launder them at least three times a week.

Plastic scrubbers: Bacteria may not attach as easily to plastic as they do to sponges and dishrags, says Stuart Levy, MD, a professor of molecular biology and microbiology at Tufts University School of Medicine. Rinse thoroughly and air-dry before storing.

Paper towels: They are better than dishrags or sponges for wiping up germy messes. To reduce the environmental toll, choose an unbleached, 100 percent recycled variety.

Disinfectants: Use these to clean a countertop where you've worked with raw meat or poultry. Look for an EPA registration number on the label, which means the product really kills germs. But be picky: You can't sterilize air, so skip aerosol disinfectants.

Shelf liner: Use self-sticking paper that won't let water leak through. If something does drip and mold develops, it's easier to replace liner than it is to replace the shelf.

Garbage can with lid: The lid is key. It contains odors and keeps any mold spores on your trash from escaping and starting a colony in the cabinet. Empty the bag daily.

Toss

Oven cleaner: The chemicals in it can burn skin on contact, and the fumes hurt airways. Instead, sprinkle a generous amount of baking soda in a cool oven and spray with a mix of water and some liquid soap to dampen. Scrub with fine steel wool.

"It takes a little longer, but it's as effective as chemicals," says Kevin Kennedy, a certified indoor environmental consultant in Kansas City, Missouri.

Antibacterial soap: Antibacterials offer imperfect protection against illness because they don't kill viruses, says Kenneth Rosenman, MD, a professor of medicine at Michigan State University. And some people are allergic; for them, antibacterials in household cleaners may cause asthma. Experts also believe that by killing only some bacteria, these soaps give rise to more dangerous strains. For most of us, soap and water is best.

Sponges. Germs breed fast on these when wet. Also, "antibacterial" sponges aren't a good option; they're likely treated with triclosan, which is an antimicrobial that might irritate sensitive skin and may harm the environment.

IN THE MEDICINE CABINET

Yes, it's called the medicine cabinet, but you should get the medicine out of it. The humidity in your bathroom can degrade medication, warns Cynthia LaCivita, PharmD, director of education and special programs at the American Society of Health-System Pharmacists (ASHP). Move your meds to a cool, dry spot, such as the linen closet or pantry. Here's what else should and shouldn't be in the cabinet.

Keep

Pill organizer: It's an easy way to keep track of your weekly meds, and research shows it helps improve adherence to complicated drug regimens. To store meds, however, keep them in their original containers, says Kathy Besinque, PharmD, an associate professor of clinical pharmacy at the USC School of Pharmacy. That way you have access to the label information and expiration dates.

Tweezers: Clean them with rubbing alcohol before using to remove splinters, for example, and toss at the first sign of rust. No need for a supersharp pair: "You shouldn't be doing surgery at home," says Besinque. Instead, look for a flat, angled tip, which is the safest, and best for precision eyebrow plucking.

Mouthwash: Those with and without alcohol work equally well. Just be sure to check your mouthwash for the American Dental Association Seal of Acceptance label. To receive the seal, manufacturers must supply studies supporting label claims, like antigingivitis and anticavity. (For a list of products, go to ada.org/seal.)

Electric toothbrush: Power-assisted types are more effective at removing plaque than brushing by hand, says Diane Melrose, RDH, chair of dental hygienics at the University of Southern California.

Dental floss: Waxed floss slides easily between tight-spaced teeth and is gentler on gums than the unwaxed type.

OTC pain relievers: Generic acetaminophen, aspirin, and ibuprofen are as reliable as brand names. Buy a bottle you'll use up before it expires, and store it with other meds in a cool spot. Other staples: antacids, antibiotic cream, and antihistamines.

Toss

Expired drugs: Most medications (about 90 percent, according to FDA tests) still get results after their expiration dates. But since crucial meds (including insulin and nitroglycerin) lose effectiveness soon after they expire, experts say it's safest to get rid of outdated medicine, as well as any leftover prescriptions.

Ipecac. For decades, this was used to induce vomiting in poison victims, but today, experts recommend against it. There's no evidence it actually helps, and it may make you less able to tolerate other poison treatments.

Frayed toothbrush. If you prefer a regular toothbrush, change it every 3 to 4 months or as soon as the bristles start looking spread out, says Kerry Maguire, DDS, MPH, director of the professional advocacy team at Tom's of Maine. A frayed brush can damage gums and doesn't clean well.

Mercury thermometer. Break it and you can inhale vaporized mercury, a neurotoxin. Even the small amount in a thermometer can be a health risk, especially if you use a vacuum cleaner on the spill. Some pharmacies offer a safer digital model in exchange for a mercury one, says Catherine Tom-Revzon, PharmD, former clinical pharmacy manager at Children's Hospital at Montefiore in Bronx, New York. Don't just throw your mercury thermometer away. Call your local recycling center for disposal instructions.

IN THE BATHROOM VANITY

Though a spray of air freshener can make your bathroom smell like vanilla, think twice before using it. In an as yet unpublished study, 25 scented products—including air fresheners and cleaners—were found to emit a toxic chemical, says Dr. Steinemann, author of the study. Instead, place cinnamon sticks in a small basket. Here are more tips.

Keep

Hairbrush: Natural bristles remove more hair-product buildup than synthetic brushes; they're also better at spreading your own natural oil evenly along hair shafts. Clean your brush with shampoo, rinse, and air-dry.

Rubbing alcohol: It's a great antiseptic for cleaning the unbroken skin around minor cuts, scrapes, and burns. It'll hurt if applied to open wounds, though. Use soap and water instead, suggests Besinque.

Toss

Old makeup: Because of infection risk, throw away eye products—mascara, eyeliner, shadow—after 6 months of daily use. Foundation lasts for about 2 years; dry face powder and lipstick stay safe for about 3.

Chemical drain de-clogger: Most emit harmful fumes and can burn skin on contact. Safer options: a plunger (and a little elbow grease) or a declogger made from bacteria that eat the kinds of gunk that block your pipes, such as Drainbo (drainbo.com).

"Bacteria-based drain cleaners aren't speedy, but they're environmentally friendly and work well," says Kennedy.

Bathroom cleaners: Most commercial toilet bowl, tub, and tile cleaners give off nasty fumes and can be fatal if ingested. Products with a Design for the Environment label are the safest available—except for those you make yourself. First, wipe surfaces with vinegar, and then sprinkle on baking soda. Let stand for a few minutes, rub with a damp sponge, and rinse.

"Vinegar is a mild acetic acid, and when it reacts with baking soda, it can help loosen surface scum," says Kennedy.

Aerosol sprays: People who use spray cleaning products are more likely to develop asthma than those who apply cleaner directly to the surface. Choose a pump-style hairspray, too.

IN THE GARAGE CABINET

The garage may hold the most potent and hazardous products in your home; keep cabinets locked if you have children or pets. Store all potentially dangerous materials in their original containers so you can easily access any important safety information. Here's some more advice for your garage cabinet.

Keep

Boric acid: This is an effective bug killer but does not evaporate into the air or pose the more serious health risks associated with synthetic insecticides. Still, keep it out of reach of kids and pets; use it only out of their reach, such as behind appliances or under baseboards.

DEET-based insect repellent: It is considered safe by the CDC, but because liberal use may irritate your skin, experts recommend using it only if mosquitoes or ticks are multitudinous, or if Lyme disease or West Nile virus is a threat (follow directions). Otherwise, use natural repellents that are made from lemon eucalyptus.

Steel wool: Use this to plug holes where mice may be getting in. Instead of rat poison, set out traps.

Goggles: Every year, more than 1 million eye injuries occur in the home—while people are whacking weeds, say, or using bleach or other toxic liquids, according to a recent study by the American Academy of Ophthalmology. Many of these injuries could be prevented if people simply wore goggles, says Tamara Fountain, MD, spokesperson for the AAO.

Toss

Pesticides: Accidental exposure can harm a child's nervous system (or even your own if the dose is large enough). Try safer options instead. To protect your garden from plant-eating aphids, for example, drown them in water-filled yellow containers. Aphids are attracted to yellow, according to entomologists. Also consider boric acid. (See facing page.)

Ethylene glycol antifreeze: A teaspoonful spilled onto your garage floor could kill a pet that laps it up; a few tablespoons could be lethal for a child. Antifreeze made with propylene glycol is about three times less toxic than the ethylene variety; check the label before you buy.

ROOM BY ROOM MAKEOVERS

The ritual of deep cleaning doesn't just clear the cobwebs from your ceilings (and your head). It's essential for great health, too. Knowing when to pitch everything from medication to your smoke alarms helps you and your family sleep better, stay safer, heal faster, and more. The following room-by-room guide outlines some surprising expiration dates.

IN THE BEDROOM
Keep

Air conditioner: Keep air conditioners until they die. With proper maintenance, including annual servicing, a room or central air conditioner can easily run for up to 15 years, especially if you don't operate it year-round, says Bill

Harrison, president-elect of the American Society of Heating, Refrigerating, and Air Conditioning Engineers. Check the filter at least every 6 weeks, particularly in humid weather.

"If dirt covers the filter so you can't see the original material or view light through it, clean it or buy a new one," he says.

Toss

Pillows: Replace pillows every year. Hair and body oils will have soaked into a pillow's fabric and stuffing after a year of nightly use, making it a breeding ground for odor-causing bacteria and allergy-triggering dust mites. Using protectors can double the life of your pillows.

Mattress: Toss your mattress after 5 to 10 years. A good mattress lasts 9 to 10 years, according to the National Sleep Foundation, but consider replacing yours every 5 to 7 years if you don't sleep well. A study at Oklahoma State University found that most people who switched to new bedding after 5 years sleep significantly better and have less back pain.

Smoke alarm: Change smoke alarms after 10 years. After a decade of continual vigilance, a unit's sensors become less sensitive—putting you at greater risk from smoke or fire should a blaze erupt. Test smoke alarms monthly and replace batteries with new ones every year. To safeguard your family, install alarms on every level of your home, in bedrooms, and outside all sleeping areas. Scary stat: One-fifth of US homes have smoke alarms that don't work.

IN THE KITCHEN
Keep

Water filters: Keep water filters 20 percent longer than normal. "Filters that make health claims like lead removal are designed to provide a margin of safety in case they're not changed on time," says Rick Andrew, operations manager at NSF International, an Ann Arbor, Michigan–based company that tests filters. (This applies to most drinking water purifiers, including models from Culligan, Brita, and PUR.) Those equipped with expiration indicators (such as trigger lights) last 20 percent longer than their recommended life. So a filter certified to clean 100 gallons actually purifies 120. Filters without an indicator last even longer, and in fact they clean twice the number of gallons claimed.

Cutting boards: Hold on to cutting boards indefinitely. How you sanitize the board—and not its age—is what kills bugs such as E. coli and Salmonella.

"The decision to replace one is ultimately based on when you think it looks too beat up," says Brenda Wilson, PhD, an associate professor of microbiology at the University of Illinois at Urbana-Champaign. Even a board with deep cracks or grooves is safe if it's sanitized after each use. Wash the board with detergent and hot water, rinse and flood with a solution of 1 part full-strength white vinegar to 4 parts water, and let it sit for 5 minutes. Rinse with clean water, pat with a clean towel, and air-dry.

Toss

Vitamins: Replace vitamins after 2 years. Independent tests find that most nutritional supplements are good for 3 years if stored in a cool, dry place, says William Obermeyer, PhD, vice president for research at ConsumerLab.com. Because the product may have been sitting on store or warehouse shelves for a year, chuck it 2 years after purchase if there's no expiration date.

Fire extinguishers: Toss fire extinguishers every 10 years. Portable extinguishers may lose pressure over time and become ineffective—whether or not they've been triggered, says Lorraine Carli, national spokesperson for the National Fire Protection Association. If your extinguisher is rechargeable, have it serviced every 6 years or when the pressure is low. (Look for service companies in the Yellow Pages under Fire Extinguishers.)

IN THE BATHROOM
Keep

Dandruff shampoo: Hang on to dandruff shampoo for 3 years. Most medicated shampoo will stay effective at least that long if there isn't an expiration date. Adding water to an almost-empty bottle to get the last bit from the bottom dilutes preservatives and makes them less effective. Toss the remainder after several days.

Rubbing alcohol: Use rubbing alcohol until the bottle is empty. "Rubbing alcohol practically lasts forever," says Abigail Salyers, PhD, a professor of microbiology at the University of Illinois at Urbana-Champaign. Even after exposure to air, the alcohol/water solution remains stable for years, if not decades, and the alcohol kills any microbes that might get into the bottle.

Toss

Contact lens solution: Discard contact lens solution after 3 months. "Once the seal is broken, germs can contaminate bottles that are left uncapped or that lack a backflow device, increasing your risk of infection," says Louise A. Sclafani, OD, an associate professor of ophthalmology at University of Chicago Hospital. Get a new case every 3 months, too.

Toothbrush: Replace your toothbrush every 3 to 4 months. The American Dental Association recommends a 3- to 4-month rotation because frayed and worn bristles don't clean as well—leaving teeth more vulnerable to decay.

Eye makeup: Throw away eye makeup 6 months after opening. The applicators used to apply mascara, liner, and shadow are repeatedly exposed to bacteria in the air and on your lashes; after 6 months of everyday use, they can overpower the products' preservatives, says John Bailey, PhD, chief scientist at the Personal Care Products Council. Liquid products that don't touch the eyes, such as foundation, can be used for up to 2 years; dry face products like powder and lip items are generally formulated to last at least 3.

Antibacterial cream: Toss antibacterial cream after 1 year. Beyond a year, the antibiotic is probably still good, but the chemical mix in the ointment may start to go bad, which may make the product less effective.

THE WORST PLACES FOR YOUR HEALTH

Location, location, location: Store owners aren't the only ones concerned with finding the perfect spot in which to situate their stuff. Researchers in a wide variety of fields know that how you organize your environment—from where you stand in fitness class to the place you choose to store your meds—has a surprising effect on everything from your weight to your chances of staying well. In other words, when it comes to how you feel, it's not just what you do, it's where you do it. Here, surprisingly bad locales for your health—and the best places to optimize it.

The Worst Place for Your Toothbrush

On the bathroom sink

There's nothing wrong with the sink itself, but it's awfully chummy with the toilet. There are 3.2 million microbes per square inch in the average toilet bowl, according to germ expert Chuck Gerba, PhD, a professor of environmental microbiology at the University of Arizona. When you flush, aerosolized toilet funk is propelled as far as 6 feet, settling on the floor, the sink, and your toothbrush.

"Unless you like rinsing with toilet water, keep your toothbrush behind closed doors—in the medicine cabinet or a nearby cupboard," Dr. Gerba says.

The Worst Place for Your Sneakers and Flip-Flops

In the bedroom closet

Walking through your house in shoes you wear outside is a great way to track in allergens and contaminants. A 1999 study found that lawn chemicals were tracked inside the house for a full week after application, concentrated along the traffic route from the entryway. Your shoes also carry in pollen and other allergens as well.

Reduce exposure by slipping off rough-and-tumble shoes by the door; store them in a basket or under an entryway bench. If your pumps stay off the lawn, they can make the trip to the bedroom—otherwise, carry them.

The Worst Place to Try to Fall Asleep

Under piles of blankets

Being overheated can keep you from nodding off, researchers say: A natural nighttime drop in your core temperature is what triggers your body to get drowsy.

To ease your way to sleep, help your body radiate heat from your hands and feet, says Helen Burgess, PhD, assistant director of the Biological Rhythms

Research Laboratory at Rush University Medical Center in Chicago. Don socks to dilate the blood vessels in the extremities, and then take the socks off and let a foot stick out from under the blankets.

The Worst Place to Cool Leftovers

In the refrigerator

Placing a big pot of hot edibles directly into the fridge is a recipe for uneven cooling and possibly food poisoning, says O. Peter Snyder Jr., PhD, president of the Hospitality Institute of Technology and Management in St. Paul, Minnesota. Here's the reason why: It can take a long time for the temperature in the middle of a big container to drop, and this creates a cozy environment for bacteria.

You can safely leave food to cool on the counter for up to an hour after cooking, Dr. Snyder says. Or divvy up hot food into smaller containers and then refrigerate. It'll cool faster.

The Worst Place for a Workout Reminder

Stuck on your Post-It–laden fridge

A visual nudge can help, but only if you notice it, says Paddy Ekkekakis, PhD, an exercise psychologist at Iowa State University. In one study, a sign urging people to use the stairs rather than the nearby escalator increased the number of people who climbed on foot by nearly 200 percent.

Put your prompt near a decision point, Dr. Ekkekakis says—keep your pile of Pilates DVDs next to the TV; put a sticky note on your steering wheel to make sure you get to your after-work kickboxing class. Just remember: The boost that you get from a reminder is usually short-term, so you need to change the visuals often.

The Worst Place to Set Your Handbag

The kitchen counter

Your fancy handbag is a major tote for microbes: Gerba and his team's swabs showed up to 10,000 bacteria per square inch on purse bottoms—and a third of the bags tested positive for fecal bacteria! A woman's carryall gets parked in some nasty spots: on the floor of the bus, beneath the restaurant table—even on the floor of a public bathroom. Put your bag in a drawer or on a chair, Dr. Gerba says—anywhere except where food is prepared or eaten.

The Worst Place for a Nighttime Reading Light

Overhead

These fixtures put out relatively bright light—enough to significantly delay the body's secretion of melatonin, showed a 2000 study. That can wreck your night, since rising melatonin levels are a major cue for your body to prepare for sleep. A low-power light clipped to your novel will let you read but leave the room dark enough for your brain to transition into sleep mode.

Try the LightWedge ($25 to $35; lightwedge.com) or the "Itty Bitty" Slim Book Light ($40; zelco.com).

The Worst Place to Keep Medicine

The medicine cabinet

So important we'll mention it again: It's not uncommon for the temp in a steamy bathroom to reach 100°F—well above the recommended storage temperatures for many common drugs. The cutoff for the popular cholesterol drug Lipitor, for instance, is around 77°F. To stay out of the red zone, store your meds in a cool, dry place, such as in the pantry.

The Worst Place to Set Fruit before Washing It

The kitchen sink

Of all the household germ depots, the kitchen sink sees the most bacterial traffic—even more than the toilet, says Kelly Reynolds, PhD, a professor and environmental microbiologist at the University of Arizona. If the perfect berry drops while you're washing it, pop it in the trash—not your mouth.

The Worst Place for Your Coffee

The refrigerator or freezer

Think that you're preserving freshness by stashing it in the fridge? Think again. Every time you take it out of the fridge or freezer, you expose it to fluctuating temperatures, which produces condensation.

"The moisture leeches out flavor. It's like brewing a cup of coffee each time," says John McGregor, PhD, a professor in the department of food science and human nutrition at Clemson University.

The best spot to store beans or grounds: in an opaque, airtight container kept on the counter or in the pantry.

The Worst Place for Your TV

Wherever you dine

Studies show that distraction is your waistline's enemy because it can keep you from noticing how much you're eating. In a 2006 study, volunteers ate faster when watching TV than while listening to music—consuming 71 percent more macaroni and cheese when watching a show.

If you have the tube on while cooking, turn it off before dinner at the kitchen table, and avoid being tempted into eating in front of the TV in the living room. The best place for your television: up or down a flight of stairs, so you have to "work" to get a snack. You'll be much less likely to munch.

SOUND ADVICE

TOP THREE WAYS TO EXTEND YOUR LIFE

We asked Dr. David L. Katz, director of the Prevention Research Center and associate professor adjunct in Public Health at the Yale University School of Medicine in New Haven, Connecticut, one of *Prevention*'s general health advisors, what are the three most important changes to make *today* to improve—and lengthen—our lives. Here's what he urges us to do.

1. RESPECT SLEEP. Most people think of sleep as a waste of time, says Dr. Katz. But a far-reaching growing body of science proves that sleep plays a major role in mood, weight control, and even immune function. Getting 7 to 8 hours of quality sleep each night is vital to health.

2. IMPROVE A RELATIONSHIP. To paraphrase Nietzche: Life can be stressful and tasking, but a big part of dealing with it is having a why, Dr. Katz says. If you have a why, you can deal with anything. In the hustle and bustle of life, we can neglect communication and not cultivate our relationships—even the most important ones. But a loving bond is the most powerful why of all.

3. GRAB THE LEVERS OF MEDICAL DESTINY. Stop using tobacco, exercise more, and eat better, Dr. Katz says. Those three cornerstones of healthy living are at your disposal. They come down to what you do with your fingers, feet, and fork. This very short list of behaviors overwhelmingly governs our medical destinies. Tobacco use, dietary patterns, physical activity, and weight control account for an 80 percent variation in risk of all chronic disease and premature death.

   If you smoke, quit. (If you care about someone who smokes, be his or her agent of change.) Find a way to get more activity in your life. And improve your diet by eating more fresh fruits and vegetables, whole grains, and lean protein.

Part 2

WEIGHT-LOSS
WISDOM

CHAPTER 6

Start Your FAT-BURNING ENGINES!

*Our expert helps five frustrated women
beat a plateau and slim down for good*

The facts are simple: To look fit and firm at any age, you have to strength-train, says Wayne L. Westcott, PhD, exercise science coordinator at Quincy College in Massachusetts. Women lose about ½ pound of muscle a year, beginning as early as in their 20s.

But that's not inevitable. According to two studies Dr. Westcott conducted over 15 years of more than 2,800 women and men, on average, you can gain 3 pounds of muscle, lose 2 inches around your waist, and drop 4 pounds of fat—without dieting—in 10 weeks by strength-training at least twice a week. Plus, new muscle revs metabolism.

"A 3-pound muscle gain increases metabolism by about 7 percent, which translates to burning roughly 100 more calories a day," explains Dr. Westcott. The more muscle you have, the more calories you burn.

Here, Dr. Westcott (coauthor of *Get Stronger, Feel Younger*) and his associate Rita LaRosa Loud use his findings to help five women reshape their current toning routines with more impressive findings—up to 4 inches off their waists and 5 pounds down on the scale in just 8 weeks. To slim down and see results even faster, try our breakthrough tip below.

"I LIFT WEIGHTS BUT MY ARMS JIGGLE!"
—ARNESSE BROWN

Arnesse regularly worked out 4 days a week, alternating between traditional 60-minute aerobic classes and 90-minute combo ones that included cardio, weights, and ab exercises. She also did a series of upper-body moves with 6- or 8-pound dumbbells.

"I'm in my 40s and in good shape but not satisfied with my triceps," Arnesse says. "For someone who works out as much as I do, I'd like to see a little more definition."

Expert Rx: Change Things Up

Regular activity keeps you fit and healthy, but you have to keep it fresh. If you always do the same exercise with the same weight for the same number of reps, your muscles get bored.

"Muscles adapt to repetitive movements and eventually stop developing,"

HOW ANYONE CAN LOSE FIVE TIMES MORE FAT

Add interval cardio workouts, such as walking or biking, to your strength-training routine: After warming up, go at a high intensity for 8 seconds, and then recover for an equal amount of time at a slow pace; repeat. Do these intervals 3 days a week for 20 minutes and you can lose 5 pounds versus 1 pound if you did a 40-minute steady-pace workout for the same number of days, according to recent research.

says Dr. Westcott. To help Arnesse bust her plateau, he suggested challenging her muscles with the following strategies.

Mix single- and multimuscle moves. To tone a specific area, your workout should include exercises that isolate a trouble spot (single-muscle moves) and those that also work the surrounding muscles. You'll get better results, says Dr. Westcott, because you're still training the target area but not overloading it to the point of injury.

Practice the 6-second rep. Lift for 2 counts, lower in 4. That's the breakdown that challenges you the most, says Dr. Westcott. The reason: Your muscles are strongest during the eccentric contraction, or lowering phase. "Slowing down this part of the exercise makes your muscles work significantly harder," he says.

Sample Workout

One set of 10 reps, 2 or 3 times per week

What you need: Bench and set of dumbbells

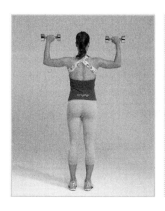

⊙ OVERHEAD PRESS

FIRMS SHOULDERS, ARMS

Stand with feet hip-width apart, abs tight, heels pressed into floor with dumbbells just above shoulders, palms facing forward and elbows out to sides (shown left). Lift dumbbells straight up in 2 counts, keeping elbows slightly bent, then slowly lower to start position in 4 counts.

CHEST PRESS

FIRMS CHEST, SHOULDERS, TRICEPS

Lie faceup on bench, feet on floor, holding dumbbells with arms extended above chest and palms forward. Bend elbows out to sides as you lower weights toward chest in 4 counts (don't let elbows drop below bench). Press weights up to start position in 2 counts.

BENT-OVER ROW

FIRMS UPPER BACK, BICEPS

Kneel with right knee and right hand on bench, left foot on floor, and abs tight with back straight from top of head to butt. Hold dumbbell in left hand with arm extended under shoulder, palm facing bench. Pull elbow toward ceiling in 2 counts as you lift weight to rib cage, then lower to start position in 4 counts.

STANDING TRICEPS EXTENSION

FIRMS TRICEPS

Stand with feet hip-width apart, abs tight, heels pressed into floor, and arms extended above head holding dumbbells with palms facing each other. Lower dumbbells straight behind head in 4 counts, keeping elbows close to ears; lift up to start position in 2 counts.

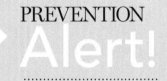

PREVENTION Alert!

10 SIMPLE RULES FOR WEIGHT LOSS

When it comes to losing weight, tried-and-true strategies work, period. Obese adults who were given a pamphlet with 10 basic rules were motivated enough to lose 4 pounds in 8 weeks. Follow them all, and you could shave off up to 900 calories a day, study authors say—enough to lose nearly 15 pounds in the same amount of time.

- Eat your meals on a regular schedule.
- Choose low-fat foods.
- Wear a pedometer and walk 10,000 steps a day.
- Pack healthy snacks.
- Check the fat and sugar content on food labels.
- Portion wisely and skip seconds (except vegetables).
- Stand for 10 minutes every hour.
- Avoid sugary drinks.
- Turn off the television while you eat.
- Eat at least 5 servings of fruits and veggies daily.

Arnesse's Results

"I was excited to lose almost 5 pounds in 6 weeks, but the best part is there's a noticeable change in my upper body. When I'm wearing a T-shirt, I can see the difference in the backs of my arms. The muscles aren't bulky at all; they just look nice."

"I WALK BUT I'M STILL FLABBY"
—MARY GODLEY, 39

Although Mary logged 30 to 45 minutes of brisk walking two or three times a week, she still couldn't get rid of her postbaby flab more than a year after the birth of her daughter.

"I used to wear formfitting shirts without feeling self-conscious," she says. "Now, I always choose loose clothing and cringe if I have to put on anything without sleeves."

Expert Rx: Add Strength-Training

Cardio exercises, such as walking and jogging, are great for burning fat and keeping your heart and lungs healthy, explains Dr. Westcott, but they do little to build the muscle that gives you a toned look. For that, you need to lift weights. Here's how to get started.

Use heavy-enough weights. The amount you lift should be light enough for you to complete at least 8 reps of an exercise using good form, but heavy enough that by the 12th rep, your muscles are so fatigued you can't imagine doing another one.

Trade dumbbells for a weighted ball. Mary had tried lifting weights in the past, but she gave it up because it was "time-consuming and boring." To spark her interest, Dr. Westcott created a routine using a weighted medicine ball (sporting goods stores; $25 to $35).

"It's less intimidating than dumbbells, and many people find that it feels more like play than exercise," Dr. Westcott says. Holding the ball with both hands is also simpler than trying to synchronize dumbbell movements with each hand.

One set of 8 to 12 reps, 3 times per week
What you need: weighted ball

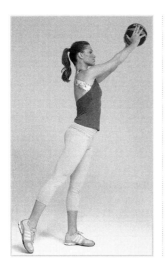

⊘ KNEE LIFT WITH PULL-DOWN

FIRMS SHOULDERS, ARMS, OBLIQUES, BUTT, THIGHS

Stand tall with feet staggered, left leg about 1 foot in front of right, abs in, and holding medicine ball with both hands over left shoulder (shown left). Slowly pull ball diagonally across body toward right hip, twisting right, while lifting right knee toward left shoulder. Return to start and repeat. Do all reps on left leg, then switch sides and repeat.

STEP HOP

FIRMS ABS, BUTT, LEGS

Stand tall, feet hip-width apart, abs in, and knees slightly bent. Hold medicine ball in front of belly, elbows close to sides. Keeping ball steady, hop to right, balancing on right leg while lifting left knee up to touch ball. Pause 1 count, then hop onto left foot, balancing as you lift right knee up to ball. Pause 1 count. (That's 1 rep.)

ARM AND LEG SWING

FIRMS SHOULDERS, OBLIQUES, BUTT, INNER AND OUTER THIGHS

Stand tall, feet hip-width apart, abs in, and knees slightly bent. Hold medicine ball in front of belly, elbows close to sides. In a slow, controlled motion, lift left leg across right while bringing medicine ball toward left side of body; keep torso facing forward. Pause 1 count, squeezing inner thighs. Then slowly swing left leg out to left side while bringing ball to right side of body. Pause 1 count, contracting outer thigh and glutes. (That's 1 rep.) Do all reps on right leg, then switch sides and repeat. Tip: Try not to use momentum or arch lower back.

CRUNCH ROLL

FIRMS ABS

Lie faceup, knees bent, and feet flat on floor. Hold medicine ball on belly. Exhale as you lift head, neck, and shoulders off floor, rolling ball up thighs toward knees. Pause at top for 1 count; inhale and roll ball back down thighs to return to start.

Mary's Results

"The moves were new to me, so I didn't get bored, and in just 3 weeks, I noticed my pants felt looser. After 8 weeks, I lost 4 inches off my waist and dropped almost 5 pounds."

"I DON'T SEE RESULTS WITH STRENGTH-TRAINING CLASSES"—TARA HEALY, 45

When Tara began losing muscle tone about 5 years ago, she started taking an hour-long sculpting class at her gym three times a week using hand weights and doing lots of reps. But after a year and a half, she saw minimal, and then eventually no more, improvement.

Expert Rx: Focus on Quality, not Quantity

Doing numerous reps with lighter weights doesn't have the same muscle-building effect as doing fewer reps with a heavy weight, says Dr. Westcott. Tara can do the same moves from class, but following these tips.

PREVENTION Alert!

BANK ON WEIGHT LOSS

Still struggling to shed pounds? Have your spouse offer you a cash prize. A 3-month study by the Research Triangle Institute in North Carolina found that dieters given just $14 per downtick in their body weight percentage lost a pound more each month than those not offered any incentive. They were also more than five times as likely to shed 5 percent of their body weight as those who weren't paid to slim down.

Practice proper form. When you churn through dozens of reps, you might start to get tired and sloppy. Instead, focus on every stage of the exercise. No bouncing, slumping, or jerking allowed.

Lift more. To keep muscles challenged, gradually increase both the reps and weight over several weeks. Choose a weight you can lift for 12 reps with proper form. Then move up to a heavier weight next time (say, from 5 to 7 pounds). Start with 8 reps at the new weight, and slowly work back up to 12 reps; then bump up the weight again.

Tara's Results

"After 6 weeks, I lost 3 inches around my waist. I developed bad habits in class, but the form fixes were worth the effort because I feel and look more toned. My new routine takes less time, and I get better results."

"CRUNCHES AND YOGA AREN'T FLATTENING MY BELLY"—SHEILA NUTT, 59

Ever since Sheila hit her mid-40s, she has watched the pounds gradually pile around her middle—even with her committed routine of 100 crunches and yoga stretches, three mornings a week.

Expert Rx: Target All Ab Muscles

Crunches are great to shape the abs, but you also have to work the hip flexors and obliques to really tone your midsection. Here's how to tweak the crunch, plus some new toning tricks.

Slow down. "When you speed through any exercise, your body's momentum propels the movement, so the muscles don't have to work as hard and you don't get results," says Dr. Westcott. Each crunch should take a full 7 seconds—3 seconds to lift, a 1-second hold at the top, and 3 seconds to lower.

Do strength-building yoga moves. Poses that require you to support your entire body weight, such as the boat or plank, might be among the best at strengthening your core because you have to engage your deep abdominal muscles, often for 30 to 60 seconds.

Two sets; 4 reps, work up to 16 (except half boat and plank), every other day

What you need: cushioned surface

KNEE-UP CRUNCH

FIRMS ABS AND HIP FLEXORS

Lie faceup, legs extended, heels on floor, and hands behind head. Lift shoulders, point right elbow forward, and raise right knee to meet elbow; keep left leg on floor. Repeat on other side. (That's 1 rep.)

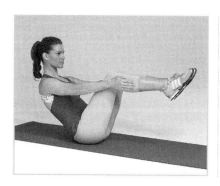

< HALF BOAT

FIRMS ABS

Sit on floor, knees bent, and feet down. Lean back, engaging abs, and lift feet, keeping back straight and knees bent with shins parallel to floor (shown left). Reach forward with hands, keeping arms at shoulder level. Balance for 30 counts.

PUSH-PULL

FIRMS ABS AND OBLIQUES

Lie faceup, hands behind head, and legs extended 45 degrees off floor. Lift shoulders and twist upper body to right, bringing right knee toward left elbow; then left knee to right elbow. (That's 1 rep.)

PLANK

FIRMS ABS, LOWER BACK

Lie facedown, resting on forearms, hands flat. Push off floor; keep weight on arms and toes. Keep back in a straight line from head to heels. Hold for 30 counts.

Sheila's Results

"Once I started slowing down my crunches and adding the other ab moves to my routine, I felt the muscles all around my midsection working. Within 3 weeks, I could button my favorite pants again. After 6 weeks, my waistline shrank 1½ inches."

"I'M TOO BUSY TO WORK OUT!"
—KELLY FLEMING, 44

With three children under age 11, Kelly found it to be very hard to maintain a regular exercise routine.

"I'd plan to go to the gym on a Saturday morning but end up having to drive one of the kids someplace instead," she says. When she did work out, she'd often overdo it to make up for missed sessions and then wouldn't feel like going back for weeks.

Expert Rx: Do Shorter, Regular At-Home Workouts

To keep fit, Kelly needs to have more consistency, not the occasional all-or-nothing routine.

"Her marathon exercise sessions may actually have interfered with her progress," says Dr. Westcott. You need time to recover after weight training, which causes microscopic tears in muscle tissue that your body then rebuilds. "One extra-long workout can deplete your energy for days, energy your body needs to get stronger," Dr. Westcott says. To create a routine to fit any busy schedule, he suggests the following time-saving tips.

Stick to 20-minute strength-training sessions. "According to our studies, it's just enough time to work every body part and make a difference, but not so much that it feels like a burden," says Dr. Westcott.

Make basic moves harder. You don't need equipment to challenge your muscles. Simple variations or a shift in body position can either work the target muscle harder or bring more muscles into play. (See pages 89–91 for some ideas to "make it harder.")

Do these exercises as a circuit, 10 reps per move, going from one exercise to the next without taking a rest; complete the circuit 3 times through. Do this circuit 2 or 3 times per week.

What you need: seat, cushioned surface

STEP-UP

FIRMS BUTT, LEGS

Stand facing sturdy seat, feet together, and arms at sides. Place right foot up on seat, knee bent 90 degrees. Pushing into right heel, step left foot onto seat next to right. Slowly step left foot down, then right. Repeat, placing left foot on seat and stepping up with right. (That's 1 rep.)

MAKE IT HARDER: Add a high knee lift at the top of your step.

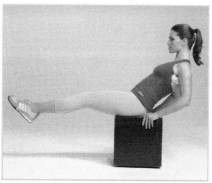

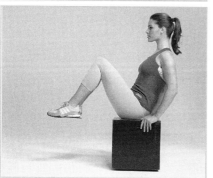

< KNEE-UP

FIRMS ABS, HIP FLEXORS

Sit on edge of seat, abs in, and legs together. Grip edge of seat behind hips and lean back slightly, extending legs straight in front of you (shown left). Slowly lift knees toward chest and exhale (shown below); inhale as you straighten legs back to starting position, but keep feet off floor.

MAKE IT HARDER: Do the move on the floor and lift your hands.

PUSH-UP

FIRMS CHEST, ARMS, ABS

Begin in a modified push-up position, hands on floor under shoulders and knees down, forming a straight line from head to hips. Lower chest toward floor, bending elbows 90 degrees; hold for 1 count and press up to start.

MAKE IT HARDER: Do a full push-up with straight legs.

SQUAT

FIRMS THIGHS, BUTT

Stand with feet hip-width apart, and arms at sides. Bend knees 90 degrees as if sitting in a chair behind you; keep weight over heels (lift arms forward to help you counterbalance). Hold for 1 count and squeeze glutes as you stand back to start position.

MAKE IT HARDER: Jump up between each rep, landing in squat position.

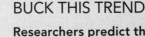

PREVENTION Alert!

BUCK THIS TREND

Researchers predict that 75 percent of US adults will be overweight by 2015. The good news: This trend is reversible. Data from the National Weight Control Registry tells us that successful "losers" share four common behaviors.

- **90 percent exercise, on average, about 1 hour per day**
- **78 percent eat breakfast every day**
- **75 percent weigh themselves at least once a week**
- **62 percent watch less than 10 hours of TV per week**

A BMI of 25 to 29.9 is defined as overweight; 30 or more, as obesity. To check yours, visit prevention.com/weightloss.

YOUR FAT-BURNING GAME PLAN

Follow this simple plan to get the scale moving in a downward direction. Is your scale stuck? Sometimes it just takes some simple changes to get the scale moving in a downward direction. Here are a few techniques to try. Incorporate as many of these into your life as you can.

Every Day

- **Wear a pedometer.**
- **Eat five minimeals (300 calories each).**
- **Log your food choices before you eat.**
- **Drink at least six 8-ounce glasses of cold water.**

Three Times a Week

- **Lift weights, doing multimuscle moves such as chest presses.**
- **Rest no more than 20 seconds between sets while strength-training.**

Whenever You Exercise

- **Snack before your workout.**
- **Schedule exercise before a meal so you eat within a half hour of finishing your workout.**
- **Track your heart rate during cardio.**

Weekly

- **Change one move in your workout routine every Monday.**
- **Plan an active outing such as hiking.**

DIPS

FIRMS TRICEPS

Sit on edge of seat and grip front edge with hands shoulder-width apart. Extend legs straight in front of body with heels on floor. Lift hips forward, keeping body close to seat. Exhaling, slowly bend elbows 90 degrees behind you, lowering hips toward floor. Inhaling, push back up and repeat; don't lock elbows at the top.

MAKE IT HARDER: Lift one leg for first 5 reps; switch legs for second 5 reps.

Kelly's Results

"Working out doesn't seem like a chore anymore. I saved so much time, and I felt firmer in just 2 weeks. I was even more thrilled to lose 2½ pounds and ½ inch off my waist after 6 weeks."

CHAPTER 7

EAT FOR A SLIM BELLY

Boost the benefits of your workout and burn more fat, faster, with these smart food choices and simple food swaps

It'll come as no surprise that what you eat—and how much of it—plays a huge role in how much you weigh. What might be more surprising is how just a few additions to your regular diet, and a few more substitutions, can make a dramatic difference.

WHAT TO EAT FOR A SLIM BELLY

Add the following to your daily diet, and you can shed about 10 pounds over the course of a year. Simple!

Water with Lemon

A California study of 240 women found that dieters who replaced their sweetened drinks with water lost an average of 3 pounds more a year than those who didn't. Subjects who sipped more than 4 cups of water a day lost 2 additional pounds, compared with those who drank less. Plus, the phosphoric acid in soda may contribute to bone loss—and osteoporosis—by changing the acid balance in your blood.

High-Fiber Granola Bars

A small British study found that women who eat a fiber-rich, high-carb breakfast burn twice as much fat during workouts later in the day as those who eat more refined (lower-fiber) foods. Try a granola bar with at least 4 grams of fiber, like Kashi, instead of the typical bar that contains just a single gram.

Refined carbs spike your insulin levels, limiting your body's ability to use fat as fuel, explains Lisa Dorfman, RD, adjunct professor at the University of Miami.

Ground Flaxseed

Flaxseed is rich in fiber and healthy fats, which help stabilize blood sugar, so you're less likely to binge. Some research suggests flax can also help soothe symptoms of hormone swings because it's high in plant estrogens.

Ground seeds are easier to digest. Sprinkle them over cereals, soups, or salads; add them to smoothies; or substitute 1 cup of ground flaxseed for ⅓ cup canola, corn, or other oil or shortening in muffins and cookies. Note: Lower oven temperature slightly, since baked goods brown faster with flax.

Walnuts

Instead of snacking on some chips, open up a bag of nuts: Walnuts are rich in omega-3 fatty acids, which may keep you feeling fuller longer.

In a 1-year study of people with diabetes who were following a low-fat diet, Australian researchers discovered that those who included 8 to 10 walnuts a day lost more weight and body fat. The subjects also reduced their insulin levels, which helps keep fat storage in check.

Hot Sauce

Forget bland condiments. To burn fat, spice things up. In a study of 36 men and women, Australian researchers found that after a spicy meal, levels of insulin—the hormone that triggers body fat storage—were lowered 32 percent.

One theory: Capsaicin, the chemical that gives chiles their fire, may improve the body's ability to clear insulin from the bloodstream after you eat, so you're more likely to burn fat following a meal spiked with chile peppers than after one that isn't packing heat.

Cinnamon

Sweeten your oatmeal or frothy coffee drinks with this sweet spice instead of sugar (16 calories per teaspoon) and you can save a couple hundred calories a week, enough to shed 2 to 3 pounds in a year without doing anything else.

You'll also be doing your heart a favor as protective estrogen levels decline: Pakistani researchers found that $1/2$ teaspoon of cinnamon a day could lower heart-damaging cholesterol by 18 percent and triglycerides by 30 percent.

Salmon

Just 3 ounces of canned salmon delivers 530 IU (more than the Daily Value) for vitamin D and 181 milligrams of calcium, a power-packed nutritional combination that may be just what your waistline needs as you get older.

In a 7-year study of more than 36,000 women ages 50 to 79, researchers at Kaiser Permanente found that those who took both calcium and vitamin D supplements gained less weight after menopause than those who took a placebo. Other research shows that without enough vitamin D, our appetite-regulating hormone leptin can't do its job. Other fatty fish choices include tuna, sardines, and mackerel.

MAKE THESE SWAPS FOR A SLIM BELLY

All you need are a few simple changes to cut 500 calories a day. That adds up to about a pound of weight loss each week. Many of the healthier alternatives also contain monounsaturated fatty acids (MUFAs)—such as olive oil or nuts—and whole grains. Studies show that both are powerful belly flatteners. And they're more satiating than saturated fats and refined grains, so you feel satisfied with less food. That's why some of the food swaps are smaller portions. For more calorie-cutting ideas, go to prevention.com/100calories.

INSTEAD OF . . .	CHOOSE . . .	CALORIES SAVED
Beverages		
16 oz latte	12 oz latte made with fat-free milk	120
16 oz soda	Water with a squeeze of lemon	180
16 oz Iced Mocha Frappuccino	16 oz iced coffee with fat-free milk	270
Iced tea with 2 tsp sugar and lemon	Iced tea with a squeeze of orange and lemon	30
1 c juice	½ c juice mixed with ½ c sparkling water	60
4 oz white or red wine	2 oz white or red wine with 2 oz sparkling water	50
16 oz beer	12 oz light beer	100
12 oz coffee with 2 Tbsp cream	12 oz coffee with ¼ c fat-free milk	20
Dairy and Eggs		
¼ c grated Cheddar cheese	1 Tbsp Parmesan cheese	90
½ c grated whole mozzarella	½ c reduced-fat mozzarella	85
½ c cottage cheese	½ c 1% fat cottage cheese	35
8 oz 2% milk	8 oz fat-free milk	50
2 lg eggs	3 lg egg whites	95
½ c whole milk ricotta cheese	½ c part-skim ricotta cheese	45
Snacks and Sweets		
Chocolate chip cookie, 4" diameter	4 1" squares of dark chocolate	180
1 c potato chips (about 15)	2 c air-popped popcorn	95
Tortilla chips, 1 oz bag	Baked tortilla chips, 1 oz bag	50
Snickers candy bar	Luna bar (flavor, your choice)	85
1 oz bag pretzels (about 10)	½ oz bag whole grain pretzels	55
½ c Peanut M&M's	½ c unshelled pistachio nuts	90
1 c fruit-on-the-bottom yogurt	½ c diced strawberries with ½ c fat-free vanilla yogurt	105
Grains and Carbs		
Blueberry muffin	Whole grain English muffin spread with 1 Tbsp blueberry fruit spread	270
Plain bagel	½ whole wheat bagel	125
2 slices white bread	1 slice whole wheat bread	90
½ c granola	½ c oatmeal	125

INSTEAD OF . . .	CHOOSE . . .	CALORIES SAVED
Grains and Carbs (continued)		
2 frozen waffles	1 whole grain frozen waffle	130
2 pancakes	1 whole grain pancake	75
1 c corn flakes cereal	½ c bran flakes cereal	40
1 c spaghetti with ½ c meat sauce	½ c whole wheat spaghetti, ¼ c sliced mushrooms, ½ c marinara sauce	160
1 c rice with 2 tsp butter	½ c brown rice with ½ c mixed frozen vegetables and 1 tsp olive oil	65
Hamburger bun	Whole grain pita	55
1 c mashed potatoes	½ lg plain baked potato	100
Flour tortilla (10" diameter)	Whole wheat tortilla (8" diameter)	80
8 Ritz crackers	4 low-fat Triscuit crackers	60
Protein		
3 oz chicken breast with skin	3 oz skinless chicken breast	30
3 oz New York strip	3 oz filet mignon	60
3 oz rib eye	3 oz tuna steak	55
3 oz top sirloin	3 oz salmon	95
3 oz beef meat loaf	3 oz turkey meat loaf	115
3 oz roast beef lunchmeat	3 oz chicken lunchmeat	75
3 oz ground beef patty	3 oz lean ground turkey patty	85
4 oz pork chop	3 oz pork tenderloin	100
2 slices bacon	2 slices turkey bacon	25
1 c refried beans	½ c pinto beans	135
Condiments		
2 Tbsp cream cheese	⅛ mashed avocado with lemon juice and a dash of salt and pepper	55
1 Tbsp butter	1 tsp olive oil	60
¼ c ranch dip for veggies	¼ c hummus	190
¼ c maple syrup	2 Tbsp apricot fruit spread	130
2 Tbsp peanut butter	1 Tbsp all-natural peanut, almond, cashew, or other nut butter	85
¼ c blue cheese dressing	Balsamic vinaigrette made with 1 Tbsp flaxseed oil and 1 Tbsp balsamic vinegar	175

CHAPTER 8

THE FAITH TO LOSE

Spirituality was the secret that helped these women break the cycle of emotional eating and drop stubborn pounds

They ate when they were stressed. They ate when they were lonely or frustrated. Then the guilt set in—for breaking the latest attempt at a diet, for losing the power struggle with a craving. It's an unhealthy pattern familiar to the women on these pages, and one to which many of us can relate.

So what makes us stop relying on food as a crutch and start taking control of

---

HOW YOU CAN DO IT!

Get inspired and meet more women who achieved their weight loss goals, including one reader who lost 130 pounds through faith, at prevention.com/dietsuccess.

our choices? Counseling might help some; others may need a disciplined eating plan. For these three women, the answer was faith. They share how their spirituality gave them strength to cultivate healthier habits and shed pounds for good.

"I GOT HEALTHY ON THE INSIDE"
KIMBERLY FLOYD, 43, FAIRBURN, GEORGIA

Pounds lost: 85
Height: 5'4"
Weight then: 240 pounds
Weight now: 155 pounds

Kimberly Floyd knew how to lose weight: She studied nutrition and worked as a registered nurse for almost a decade. Kimberly had reason, too: High blood pressure and stroke runs in her family. Yet when on break at the hospital, she would often down a burger and fries, and she grew to 240 pounds.

Then one evening in December 2003, when Kimberly was only 38, she had severe chest pain.

"I realized then this was not how I was supposed to live," she says. Though she first became a Christian in her mid-20s, that moment redefined her faith. "I felt like God has a purpose for my life, and I had to find strength to fulfill it." She started reading the Bible and praying daily. Instead of focusing on shedding excess fat, she told herself: "My body is the temple of the Holy Spirit, and I'll do what it takes to stay healthy." With that, making healthful choices became much easier. She swapped fast food for whole foods and added a daily walk to her routine. In a year and a half, she lost 85 pounds.

Kimberly was so inspired and motivated that she began her own Christian weight-loss–coaching program called Take Back Your Temple.

"My message is about taking responsibility and making the most of all the gifts God has given you," she says. "When you see your body as sacred, your desire to care for it intensifies."

My Faith Helps Me . . .

See the big picture: "Praying and being grateful every day gives me emotional stability and a greater perspective on life. Daily challenges don't throw me off the way they once did, and that helps me make wiser choices," Kimberly says.

Expert Tips

"Mindset is huge in terms of weight loss," says Keecha Harris, DrPH, RD, president of a health consulting firm in Birmingham, Alabama. "You have to stay positive, and that's why faith is so powerful. It's based in something good and hopeful." Here's how to stay in that frame of mind.

Set small goals. Aim to lose 1 pound this week, run $\frac{1}{2}$ mile longer next week, or switch to fat-free milk in your coffee. Attainable mini-goals keep you focused and give you a sense of progress.

Think total-body health. When you eat right or work out, you have more energy and feel happier. Noticing—and appreciating—those benefits, too, will help you stay even more motivated.

"I FOUND PURPOSE IN MY WEIGHT LOSS"
ABBY MELOY, 46, LAKE CITY, FLORIDA

Pounds lost: 56
Height: 5'8"
Weight then: 216 pounds
Weight now: 160 pounds

As senior pastor, Abby Meloy couldn't say no when parishioners asked her to organize a weight loss group at their church.

"I was hesitant because I had failed at many diets in the past," says Abby, whose weight had reached more than 200 pounds. "But I knew I wasn't setting the right example for my congregation, so I gave it a shot."

Abby started a chapter of a national Christian health program called First Place at her church. The Bible-based plan focuses on improving all areas of life—physical, spiritual, and emotional. Abby kept a food journal, balanced her meals, and committed to a daily exercise routine. Soon, she led weekly prayer groups to help empower members to overcome temptation. In the first 13 weeks, Abby dropped 27 pounds.

"When I started seeing results and others came to me for advice, my diet became about something more," she says. "If I continued to succeed, I could help others do the same. That was my motivation."

Surrounded by trusted parishioners, Abby acquired the confidence to explore the real reasons she overate, which included the stress of serving as a pastor. Now when she feels the compulsion to eat to quell her anxiety, she prays or takes a walk to clear her mind.

"If I'm still hungry afterward, I'm in a better place mentally to make a healthy choice," she says. And if she does indulge, she tries not to be too hard on herself. "I think, 'God forgives me, so why shouldn't I forgive myself?'—and then I'm right back on track."

My Faith Helps Me . . .

Find motivation: "When losing weight stopped being about me, me, me, and became about setting a good example—that's when I knew I'd be successful," Abby says.

Expert Tips

"Being a leader keeps you accountable," says Jeannie Moloo, RD, a spokesperson for the American Dietetic Association. "And that has a powerful impact on your behavior." Here are some ways to foster that sense of responsibility.

Consider yourself a role model. Set an example for your family and friends. How you act makes a lasting impression.

Team up. Working toward your goal with another person can provide extra support and inspiration.

"I MADE PEACE WITH FOOD"
JACKIE HALGASH, 54, WARRINGTON, PENNSYLVANIA

Pounds lost: 100
Height: 5'7"
Weight then: 245 pounds
Weight now: 145 pounds

Church was one of the last places Jackie thought she'd go to lose weight. Though she was raised as a Catholic, she never considered herself overly religious. Still, when a friend suggested she try a faith-based diet program, she agreed. Her weight had reached 245 pounds; she felt like she had no other place to go.

In 2002, Jackie signed up for a Catholic plan called the Light Weigh. Its message: Seek comfort in God, not food. That's what hit home for Jackie: "I'd gorge on cookies when I was sad, and it didn't help," she recalls. Through Bible study classes and videos, she figured out that she needed something more profound to feel at peace.

"It's like I had a spiritual 'hole' in my heart," explains Jackie. "I tried to fill it with food but never felt content. When I turned to prayer, I felt complete." One basic lesson she learned: Eat when you're hungry; stop when you're full. "We were given hunger cues for a reason," she says.

If she's tempted to eat more, Jackie thinks of giving up the excess food as a sacrifice for someone else—her children or the patients in the hospital where she works. "Cutting portions is easier when it's an act of love," she says. Within 18 months, Jackie lost 100 pounds—and she has maintained it since.

My Faith Helps Me . . .

Stop judging foods: "I used to think if I ate salad, I was being good; if I ate ice cream, I was bad. Now, food is simply food. There are no more moral consequences to eating," Jackie says.

Expert Tips

Follow hunger cues and control portions—both are key to losing weight, says Moloo. Here are some tips to stay on track.

Take five. When you have a craving, wait a few minutes before you eat. A change of pace or a couple of deep breaths may also help it pass.

Eat in slow motion. Put your fork down after each bite and chew your food thoroughly (and swallow) before picking it up again. This makes you more conscious of when you're full.

CHAPTER 9

The Overweight
DEBATE

*Has science overemphasized the danger of
a few extra pounds? Our writer Sarah Mahoney
explains what the latest firestorm among
researchers means for you*

Eight months ago, while traveling on business, I went to see a doctor for a minor issue. After taking care of it, she scanned my chart. "Have you considered going on a diet?" she asked. "Your weight puts you at a higher risk of heart disease and diabetes." Ouch! Blushing, I promised to follow up with my doc at home and hightailed it to my hotel, where I spent the rest of the day pacing between the full-length mirror and the jumbo bag of cashews in my purse.

It's not that I hadn't considered losing weight. I was sure I was too fat when I went to college at 113 pounds, and in my mid-30s when I weighed 140. What's different is that now, at 158, I'm clinically overweight. Experts define it as having a body mass index (BMI) between 25 and 29.9, and at 5-foot-4, mine is 27—not even borderline.

On the brighter side, I live a healthier life than the average Jane. I exercise almost every day—walks, weights, yoga. My diet is packed with fruit, vegetables, and whole grains—albeit in larger portions than a dietitian might advise. I traded the high stress of New York City for rural Maine, where rush hour involves dogs, family, and wild turkeys outside my window. I knit. I garden. Heck, I even meditate. Doesn't any of this count? Or is that darned scale the only thing anyone cares about?

BEYOND THE BMI

Turns out, I'm not the only one asking these questions. In fact, in light of several new studies, experts are divided on the danger posed by excess weight, especially if the person is, like me, generally healthy and fit. Much of the research linking excess weight and an increased risk of diabetes, heart disease, and cancer, among other chronic diseases (the list goes on and on), has been done on people who are obese, with a BMI of 30 or more. When the merely overweight folks are separated out, the health risks drop and sometimes even disappear.

"Being overweight may not be associated with any risk of heart disease," says Robert Eckel, MD, a professor of medicine at the University of Colorado and past president of the American Heart Association.

Recently, researchers from the CDC and the National Cancer Institute (NCI) caused waves in the medical community with a report analyzing the death records of 37,000 adults. Although obese folks had a greater risk of dying from cancer or heart disease, those who were simply overweight had, surprisingly, no greater risk than normal-weight people. Even more amazing, the findings suggested that being overweight may actually protect against death from a multitude of diseases other than cancer and heart disease. The research made headlines: "Is That Spare Tire a Lifesaver?"

Critics quickly responded that the study failed to consider quality-of-life issues caused by excess pounds and didn't appropriately control for unhealthy habits like smoking, which can keep people lean but undeniably raise cancer risk. Still, it added fuel to the ongoing debate of whether losing weight is absolutely necessary to reduce disease risk if you're not obese.

However, no one's debating that weight loss can be one part of an overall disease prevention plan. But is it really the most essential first step? That depends on how many other disease risk factors you have, says Dr. Eckel. Here are some factors to consider.

Age: Anyone 45 or older is at a higher risk of diabetes, and a woman's risk of heart disease begins to rise at 55. Cancer risk also increases with age. (Talk about a midlife crisis.)

CHECK YOUR RISK FACTORS

Guidelines suggest that obese people should slim down, but experts say that overweight people may be fine, barring the risk factors listed below. If two or more of them apply to you, you need to talk with your doctor about reducing your weight by 5 to 10 percent.

HEART DISEASE RISK: That means a family history of heart disease (men having heart attacks before 55 and women before 65), stroke, or high blood pressure.

TOO LITTLE EXERCISE: If you exercise anything less than 30 minutes 4 days a week, it is simply inadequate.

DIABETES RISK: This includes a family history of the illness, as well as having had an impaired glucose test in the past.

TOO MUCH BELLY FAT: For women, having a waist measurement that is greater than 35 inches is a red flag.

MIDDLE AGE: Because anyone who is 45 years old or older is at a higher risk of diabetes, and women's risk of heart disease begins to rise at age 55, midlife is considered a risk factor all its own.

BAD BLOOD: A total cholesterol level of 200 mg/dL or more, or an HDL reading of less than 40 mg/dL, raises risk.

Family history: I always assumed that because many in my family had died from heart disease, I was in trouble.

But it turns out that what really matters is early heart disease. For men that means a heart attack before age 55 and for women, age 65. Even then, only first-degree relatives—parents, children, and siblings—are considered red flags. And while it's true that type 2 diabetes rarely occurs in people who aren't overweight or obese, the risk of developing the disease is 5 to 10 times higher if a first-degree relative has it—regardless of your weight.

As far as the big C is concerned, only about 5 to 10 percent of cancers are inherited, and those that are typically occur earlier in life. According to the American Cancer Society (ACS), most cancers are caused by gene mutations brought on by age, lifestyle, and environmental factors, such as inactivity, smoking, excessive alcohol consumption, and increased exposure to radiation or carcinogenic chemicals, among others.

In fact, researchers from Britain's Million Women Study found that 5 percent of all cancers affecting postmenopausal women in the United Kingdom are associated solely with excess body weight. Indeed, the ACS and the NCI acknowledge that while being overweight and obese are linked to an increased risk of cancer, there is limited evidence that losing pounds will reduce that risk.

Waist measurement: For women, a waistline of 35 inches or larger is a risk factor for heart disease, no matter how much you weigh or how trim your arms and legs are. And a measurement of 31.5 inches or more indicates an elevated risk of some cancers.

Fitness: Walking briskly for 30 minutes 5 days a week is enough to protect you from disease, no dieting required.

"Fitness is achievable, and may do more to improve health than simply losing weight," says Steven Blair, PED, a professor of exercise science at the University of South Carolina and a leading expert on the benefits of exercise among the overweight.

In fact, a recent study from the university tracked 2,600 people age 60 and older for a 12-year period and found that fit overweight people outlive unfit normal-weight people. (Score one for me!) However, if you're overweight and it hurts just to walk up and down stairs, weight loss may be called for. Obese women are 4 times more likely to develop knee osteoarthritis than normal-weight women.

Cholesterol and inflammation: A total cholesterol level of 200 mg/dL or more, an HDL reading of less than 40 mg/dL, or triglyceride levels above 150 mg all point to trouble. Being overweight tends to increase cholesterol, and losing weight can help lower total and LDL levels, while raising HDL levels, according to the National Heart, Lung, and Blood Institute. (So can increasing your daily activity if you're sedentary.)

Many experts feel that your rate of systemic inflammation, as defined by the results of a C-reactive protein (CRP) test, is an even stronger indicator of heart disease risk. Being overweight raises your risk of inflammation.

WEIGHING MY OPTIONS

When I returned home, I did indeed follow up with my doctor. We discussed all of this—my high BMI, cholesterol, low blood pressure, fitness level, and CRP score—and then he calculated my Framingham Risk Score, which is a measure widely used to assess a 10-year risk of heart attacks. (You can take an online version of this test at prevention.com/links.)

Thanks to no smoking, my family history, a good diet, and an active lifestyle, my risk level came up as "very low" at 1 percent. Together, we decided that I could stay, er, voluptuous and still expect to live a reasonably long and healthy life.

I should have felt vindicated, but instead I felt like a quitter. Truth was, I hated that my knees hurt after a walk and that I dreaded bathing suit season. And so I decided to slim down anyway but resolved to go about it as sensibly as I knew how, to follow the most proven weight-loss principles available.

First, I dropped my fantasy goal of 130 (last seen before getting pregnant with my now college-bound daughter). Instead, I aimed low—5 percent of my body weight, or 7 to 8 pounds. (Experts advise shooting for no more than

10 percent at a time.) If you're overweight and have numerous risk factors for chronic disease, even a loss this small can offer some protection. Bigger goals—say, fitting into your wedding dress again—may set you up for regain.

I resolved to lose no more than a pound a week, and not to panic if I lost as little as a pound every 10 days. Researchers are adamant that the changes that bring about small losses—walking 15 minutes more a day, or using fat-free milk instead of cream in coffee—are more likely to become lasting ones. I didn't exactly ban foods like butter, cheese, ice cream, and bacon, but I cut back—switching to reduced-fat alternatives and smaller portions.

I also intensified my exercise to at least an hour most days, which is what the US Dietary Guidelines recommend for weight loss. I woke up earlier, dug out my heart-rate monitor, and added jogging intervals to my walking routine. On weekends, I didn't do yoga or go on a hike; I did both.

IS WEIGHT LOSS WORTH IT?

I'm proud to say I lost 7 pounds in 4 months, and I'm fitter and stronger. My back and knees feel better; my cholesterol is a bit lower. Maintenance, though, is a daily struggle, and as the scale number rises and falls, so does my mood. I recalculated my Framingham Risk Score with my new weight—still the same 1 percent risk. Just for fun, I keyed in my dream weight of 130. Maddeningly, no change.

Still, I realized something. Even if it wasn't about my heart health or my "relative risk of mortality," it simply feels good to weigh less. I'm happy I can walk my dogs without pain, slide into my jeans without struggle, and buy a one-piece without cringing. If that's not quality of life, what is?

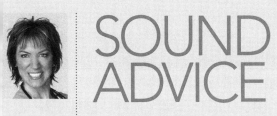

SOUND ADVICE

TO BEGIN A WEIGHT-LOSS PROGRAM

When we asked Pamela Peeke, MD, MPH, assistant clinical professor of medicine at the University of Maryland and the author of numerous best-selling books, including *Body for Life for Women* and *Fit to Live,* one of *Prevention*'s general health advisors, what she thinks are the three most important things to do before beginning a weight-loss program, here was her encouraging response.

1. **GET YOUR MIND READY.** Ask yourself: Are you ready to change? Many of us have good intentions, but readiness is a very different thing, says Dr. Peeke. Implicit in this is asking yourself if you are ready to do the work and also to adapt and adjust to whatever happens to you in life, without self-destructing and overeating.

    You also need to find *meaning* behind the readiness, she explains. That's because the meaning drives the readiness. For example, your meaning could be "I can't live one more day knowing how unhealthy I am" or "I need to get into better shape so I can play with my grandkids." Once you find the meaning for you, keep it front and center. Better yet, write it down.

2. **GET YOUR MOUTH READY.** Stick to Mother Nature's food basket, Dr. Peeke says. Eat more fresh fruits and vegetables, whole grains, and lean proteins. These are gifts from Mother Nature. Highly processed foods that come in family-sized boxes and bags are not made by Mother Nature.

3. **GET YOUR MUSCLES READY.** Find something joyful to do with your body on a regular basis, says Dr. Peeke. For example, jump rope or dance. Look for ways to turn physical activity into fun. Find some way to move your body that brings you joy. Then do it. Often.

Prevention® Exclusive
WEIGHT-LOSS
SPECIAL REPORT

TIPS, TRICKS & TECHNIQUES

by the Stars of *The Biggest Loser*

"WE LOST BIG!"

How did the stars of The Biggest Loser
drop double-digit pounds week after week?
Here's the science behind the plan.
Plus: How you can lose the weight you want

Losing 20 pounds might take the rest of us a few months. Kae Whang, a contestant on *The Biggest Loser*, did it in 1 week—breaking the female record on the hit NBC reality show. Fellow contestants Hollie Self and Isabeau Miller both shed about half that amount in the same short time.

If you watch the show, you see them test their physical and emotional limits during challenges. What you don't see is what happens the rest of the week on campus—the meal planning and calorie monitoring, the training and strengthening, the advice and support from a team of experts, all working toward the same goal: to help these participants lose weight now, keep it off later, and restore hope that they can live happy and healthy lives.

We asked three of a past season's stars, along with the show's medical and nutrition advisor, Michael Dansinger, MD, and nutritionist, Cheryl Forberg, RD, to share what it really takes to shed megapounds fast, and why the process is nothing short of life transforming. Here are eight Biggest Loser strategies that can inspire you to reach your own weight-loss goal.

BELIEVE YOU CAN DO IT

For Hollie, the show is not only changing the way she looks but also the way she looks at life: "Nothing is impossible." A little tough love from her team leader and trainer, Jillian Michaels, taught her that. "I needed someone to push me out of my comfort zone, to keep telling me, 'You can do more,'" Hollie says. Now, she's setting new goals. "I always hated running, and then one week I actually won the mini-triathlon challenge. When I get home, I want to try a real one."

Even the most confident, though, have their moments of doubt. Finding a mantra or meaningful phrase worked for Isabeau. "When I started questioning my determination, I would remember the last thing my parents said before I left for the show: 'Never, ever give up.'" And she won't until she reaches this milestone: to join her family in a 7-mile race they run every year.

DON'T FORGET TO EAT!

That means eating breakfast and lunch and dinner, plus two snacks—every single day. This isn't groundbreaking news, but according to Forberg, it's worth repeating.

"When I started working with the show, I was surprised how many contestants skipped meals," she says. That can lead to out-of-control hunger and overeating. Stick to a regular eating schedule to keep your metabolism revved, hunger satiated, and energy up. Here are some basic Biggest Loser diet principles.

Find your ideal calorie budget. Each contestant's individual calorie limit is determined by a complex formula that considers starting weight, body-fat percentage, and goal weight, says Dr. Dansinger. Kae, for example, first weighed in at 225 pounds and follows a 1,200-calorie-a-day diet, while Isabeau, who started at almost 300 pounds, eats between 1,500 and 1,600 calories daily.

At home, use this simple formula to determine your limits: If you weigh between 150 and 300 pounds, multiply your weight by 7. That number is your caloric goal each day. If you weigh more than 300 pounds, use 300 as your starting "weight." If you weigh less than 150 pounds, use 150 as your starting "weight." (Register—for free—to use My Health Trackers at prevention.com/healthtrackers to determine a good goal weight.)

Make healthy substitutions. "The quality of the calories is just as important as the quantity," says Forberg. That means choosing natural foods (such as whole grain bread) and passing up processed products (white bread). You can find a nutritious version of everything you like, says Isabeau. "At home, I had french fries with every meal. Now I have sweet potato fries. They're tasty and so much healthier." But her biggest surprise was how much she got to eat: "I'm never hungry."

Understand why. Contestants learn about nutrition so they understand why whole grain bread, for example, is better than white. (It's high in fiber, so you stay fuller longer.) "It's easier to stick to a plan that makes sense to you," says Forberg.

DO CARDIO YOU ENJOY EVERY DAY

"Before I got here, I imagined we'd start with 20 minutes one day, maybe 40 minutes the next," laughs Isabeau. "Ha!" They jumped right in, with cardio training lasting hours at a time. Should you do the same? No. Contestants are pushed to work out harder than average, but only because they are under the close supervision of trainers and a medical staff. Here's what you can do safely to reach your own fitness goal.

Shoot for 60 to 90 minutes a day. And maintain a moderately intense level. (If you're over age 50, have a chronic disease, or are at risk of one, consult your doctor before starting any plan.)

Make sure you sweat. You need to challenge yourself to get the weight-loss results you want. If your routine feels comfortable, devote a few more minutes to each workout, or add hills and/or stairs to your regular walk.

Mix it up. Repeating the same activity day after day puts you at risk of overuse injuries and could stall weight loss. Try breaking up one cardio session with a few different workouts: 20 minutes walking, 20 on the bike, 20 climbing stairs or rowing.

WEIGHT-TRAIN AT LEAST TWICE A WEEK

Strength-training helps boost your metabolism, and—as many of the contestants discovered—provides a mental lift, too.

"I came here wanting to pull my own weight, and I've done that—both literally and figuratively," says Isabeau. "I've noticed changes in my body so much more quickly since I started training, and now I can lift as much as the boys can!"

Work each muscle group at least twice a week, with 2 days off in between. For many women, that translates to 20 minutes, 4 days a week—2 days for the upper body, and 2 days for the lower body. After 2 or 3 months, they'll experience a 20 to 40 percent increase in muscular strength—the same as most men, reports the American Council on Exercise.

You don't need a trainer to get started; visit prevention.com/biggestloser for exercises and other motivational tips.

> ### MEET BIGGEST LOSER: ISABEAU 5'8"
> Before: 298 pounds; after: 246 pounds
>
> " More than anything, this process taught me to believe in myself. Instead of just talking about my dreams, I'm going to make them happen. "

TAKE ADVANTAGE OF THE EARLY MOMENTUM

Losing 20 pounds in the first week started Kae on a high note: "It inspired me to keep going and going," she says. Getting good results at first is common; use your initial enthusiasm to create healthy new habits that will see you through when your "high" wears off.

Expand your pantry. Explore the local farmer's market for something exotic (bok choy, anyone?) or sprinkle new spices on your staple meals (chili powder is a favorite in *The Biggest Loser* kitchen). The more adventurous you are now, the more new low-fat choices you'll have later so you don't get bored.

Learn new light-cooking techniques. Thumb through a cookbook or browse recipes online for some healthy tricks and then apply them to modify a favorite high-fat dish.

Find fun ways to burn calories. Take a tough yoga class, tackle a rock wall, or even sign up for a local 5-K fun run—anything you've wanted to try. You'll likely discover a new favorite workout.

EXPECT—AND PUSH THROUGH—PLATEAUS

Hollie shed 11 pounds at her first weigh-in, and she was thrilled. But the week after, she dropped only 2 pounds, and 3 the next.

"It was discouraging to work so hard and get such limited results," she says. But she kept going, reminding herself that numbers don't always reflect progress. Be patient, says Dr. Dansinger. Stick to your plan, and the scale will move again. It did for Hollie, whose weekly losses eventually crept up. If the scale stays stuck for more than 3 weeks, however, you may need to step up your exercise efforts or reevaluate your calorie intake.

BUILD A SUPPORT TEAM

One big reason contestants drop pounds so fast, says Dr. Dansinger, is the enormous team of trainers, doctors, and dietitians—not to mention the other contestants—who are there all day, every day to offer guidance and moral support. When Kae got home, her first step was to hook up with a weight-training buddy who's just as motivating as her on-set trainer, Bob Harper.

"He got to know each of us personally, but in the gym, he's dead serious," she says.

To find an exercise partner who fits your style, sign up for an online weight loss program that matches you with someone in your area, check the bulletin board at your church for walking groups, or join a running or hiking club.

FACE EMOTIONAL EATING HEAD-ON

All of the contestants had to explore their relationship with food and learn how to take control of their eating. "Some weeks are harder than others," admits Isabeau, "and when we go back home, we'll have tough weeks, too. We had to learn to work though it." Here are the favorite take-home strategies from our Biggest Loser stars.

Write down everything you eat. "It keeps you honest," says Isabeau. "Plus, I realize I don't have to cut everything I love out of my diet, like ice cream. I can have a small scoop, as long as I stay within my daily calorie allowance."

Ask yourself: Is it worth it? "I look at a piece of cake and think, Is it worth an extra hour on the treadmill? If the answer is yes, I go for it," says Kae.

Put your health first. Hollie, a teacher, found that her weight issue was an indirect result of her devotion to her students. "I focused so much on them that 'me' time was often takeout and TV. I now make my well-being a priority."

Let your success inspire you. "When contestants take control and get their health back, they often find a new person, inside and out," says Forberg. Even before the show was over, Kae knew that she'd already changed so much.

"I'm much stronger," she says—strong enough to visit her homeland of Korea, something she hasn't had the courage to do in more than 20 years. "I was too ashamed of how I looked to go see my family," she says. Even though she still hasn't reached her 110-pound goal weight, she is determined to get on that plane anyway. "I feel like I can do anything now."

"We Won the WEIGHT-LOSS MIND GAME!"

Stars of The Biggest Loser: Couples *work hard to change their bodies; they work even harder to change their mindsets. Here's how they retrain their brains for weight-loss success*

They kickbox and practice yoga. They run mini-marathons and sweat through strength-training sessions. They keep food journals, control their portions, and eat three nutritious meals, plus two snacks, a day. That's how the contestants on NBC's *The Biggest Loser: Couples* melt the pounds away. But the changes that matter most, the ones that will keep them healthy long after they leave the ranch, happen on the inside.

"Working hard to achieve a goal, such as losing weight, builds self-esteem," says Ann Kearney-Cooke, PhD, coauthor of *Change Your Mind, Change Your Body.* "You develop confidence, you become the writer of your life story—and that affects how you think, feel, and behave."

Prevention spent time on-set at *The Biggest Loser: Couples*, taking pictures and talking to some of the participants about their emotional journeys. Here, four of them—Ali Vincent, Brittany Aberle, Kelly Fields, and Jay Kruger—take us through the twists and turns, share their healthy realizations, and offer their best strategies for not just getting, but thinking thin. Plus, we offer expert tips to help you get in the weight-loss head space, too.

ALI'S STORY

Age: 33
Height: 5'5"
Weight then: 234 pounds
Weight now: 122 pounds
Lost: 112 pounds

I was once a nationally ranked synchronized swimmer and a high school cheerleader. But when I quit sports, I quit setting goals and I quit dreaming. For the past 10 years, my weight had dictated my life. It was my excuse if I got passed up for a promotion; it was the reason I was alone. I hid under my fat; it protected me from dealing with anything I did wrong or any issues I needed to work on.

When I started losing weight, it made me look at myself a little closer. I learned the only way I could move forward was to acknowledge the role I played both physically and mentally in my weight gain—and forgive myself for letting it happen. As long as I keep telling myself the truth, I'll be successful.

How I Think Thin

"I live in the moment." A journey of a thousand miles starts with one step. To me, that means every workout is a small victory, sticking to my calorie budget is another, Ali says. If I make a bad choice, that's okay; I can choose again the very next time. That gives me ownership over my life, and I know I

can do anything I want with it. And that feels good, because for a long time, I forgot I had control.

Expert Mind Tip

Start small and be realistic. Every week, set a goal for weight loss (lose 1 pound), one for cardio (run 5 extra minutes), and one for strength (do an extra set). Achieving even one is progress, and reason to feel good about yourself, says Ann Kearney-Cooke, PhD, a Cincinnati-based psychologist.

BRITTANY'S STORY

Age: 22
Height: 5'6"
Weight then: 221 pounds
Weight now: 164 pounds
Lost: 57 pounds

"You have a pretty face." That's what people always told me, but I never felt that way. I've been overweight since I was 8 years old. My parents divorced the year before. Food became my companion, a constant in my life whenever I felt lonely or sad. It's not easy for me to open up; if I don't let anyone in, I can't get hurt.

When the show started, I realized that for my team to do well, we had to get to know each other—our beliefs, our history, our goals. That experience changed me in so many ways: I faced my fears and learned to let my guard down. It made me feel good about what I can accomplish. When I look in the mirror, I can't believe that's me. I see a confident person, someone who for the first time believes she is beautiful.

How I Think Thin

"I focus on the future." Before coming to the ranch, I was diagnosed with high cholesterol and high blood pressure, Brittany says. I thought I would always be heavy, that I'd never walk with my head held up. In less than a month, my counts were back to normal. I got a second chance, and I refuse to waste it. I'll still have tough days, but I now have the tools to get through them. I plan to live life to the fullest.

Expert Mind Tip

Nurture self-esteem. It takes time to boost your body image—noticing the changes helps. Spend 5 minutes a day looking in the mirror, or measure your waist, thighs, and arms once a month and note the numbers in a journal, says Dr. Kearney-Cooke.

KELLY'S STORY

Age: 39
Height: 5'6"
Weight then: 271 pounds
Weight now: 162 pounds

I spent my adult life doing for others. I did for my ex-husband, Paul. At home, I do for my mom, and as a nurse, I do for patients. Doing for me, though—it didn't seem necessary or too important. I never felt like my own needs warranted any priority; like it was almost selfish to make time to take care of myself. But I wanted to be healthy, and I wanted to look good. It took a while for me to even feel comfortable with that, but what this experience has taught me is that I am worth it—and I deserve it, just like everybody else.

How I Think Thin

"I value my health every day." I love helping my family and doing my job, but to be a better daughter and nurse, and a better person all-around, I'll need to keep my health and well-being at the top of my to-do list, Kelly says. This means I won't always volunteer to take on extra hours at work; that also means I need to nurture my personal life. I'm stronger today than I've ever been—inside and out—so I know I can do it.

Expert Mind Tip

Lose weight for your whole life. Name five things in life you value most, such as your family or community. Now think about how getting healthy relates to those values. You'll be around longer for your family, you'll be a role model or inspiration to your community, and you'll realize the importance of taking care of you, says Dr. Kearney-Cooke.

JAY'S STORY

Age: 32
Height: 6'1"
Weight then: 293 pounds
Weight now: 190 pounds

I was the funny fat kid growing up. I'd make jokes at my own expense; it was my way of protecting myself. Decades later, not much had changed. That is, until my daughter was born with a rare overgrowth disorder; it means she'll be at least 6-foot-2. I don't want her to be overweight, as well, and go through what I did. I need to set the right example. Being heavy for so long, though, it's hard to picture yourself any differently. Even now, I don't see myself as "thin." But I look at the sizes on the clothes I'm wearing, and it blows my mind. And there's no denying how wonderful I feel inside. This is who I am now, and I plan to take advantage of it.

How I Think Thin

"Eat to live, don't live to eat." Before, I ate constantly, but now, I find other things to occupy my time, like exercise, says Jay. Going back to my old way of life would be an insult, a slap in the face to everyone who has supported me. I've come too far. I won't do that to them—or to me.

Expert Mind Tip

Know what works for you. Keep a list of your personal tips, and use it when you start to struggle. If calling a friend stopped a binge in the past, write it down; if a spoonful of peanut butter satisfied your sweet craving, note that, too, says Lyssa Menard, PhD, an assistant professor at Northwestern University.

THE BIGGEST LOSER DIET

Form a healthier relationship with food
so you, too, can eat to live, not live to eat

If you're reading this book, chances are that you're looking to change your diet. Perhaps you've tried every wacky diet on the planet—the grapefruit diet, the cabbage soup diet, the brown rice diet—only to come to the realization that while most of them work in the short term, none of those diets works for the long haul. That's because wacky, extreme diets cannot be maintained. They're either unhealthy, too limiting, too boring, too depressing, or all of the above.

So if you're looking for a plan that works, you're ready for the Biggest Loser diet. It's sensible, healthy, and flexible, and you can maintain it for the rest of your life. It's a diet that at a certain point won't feel like a diet anymore—a diet that becomes so integrated into your life and your being that it becomes your lifestyle.

Here's what you need to know about the Biggest Loser diet: It's calorie-controlled, carbohydrate-modified, fat-reduced, and high in lean protein, which controls hunger. Let's get specific. You'll get to eat three meals and two snacks every day, so you'll never be hungry or feel deprived. You can choose from an amazing, colorful variety of foods, as long as most of those foods are natural and not processed. Natural foods contribute greatly to weight loss, because they are generally lower in calories, have more fiber, and are more satisfying than processed foods.

CALORIES REALLY DO COUNT

A calorie is the measurement of how much energy a food gives your body after you eat it. You need calories to live, and if they're the right kind of calories, you live better. But if you take in more calories than you burn through daily activity and exercise, you'll gain weight—regardless of whether those calories come from "good" natural foods or "bad" processed foods. It's that simple. The formula for losing weight is even simpler: Eat less, exercise more. But how do you know how many calories you need?

Here's the easy-to-work equation we've put together to help you: If you weigh between 150 and 300 pounds, multiply your present weight by 7. That number is your caloric goal for each day on the Biggest Loser diet. If you weigh more than 300 pounds, use 300 as your starting "weight" for this formula. Likewise, if you weigh less than 150 pounds, use 150 as your starting "weight."

WHAT SHOULD YOU EAT?

To give the Biggest Losers an easy template to build their daily menus, we designed the 4-3-2-1 Biggest Loser Pyramid. The bottom, or widest tier, represents the fruits and vegetables in your diet. You should eat at least four servings daily. The next tier up represents protein foods, of which you should have three servings daily. The next tier is for whole grains, of which you should have two servings daily. And the top tier is extras, of which you can have 200 calories daily. A serving equals 8 ounces (or 1 cup), which comes out to be about the size of your hand.

Fabulous Fruits and Vegetables

On the Biggest Loser diet, fruits and vegetables are your best friends. Because these wonder foods supply the most nutrients for the fewest calories, you get to eat more of them than anything else. At least half of your daily four servings should be from vegetables; the other half should be from fruits. You might eat more than four daily servings if you wish, as long as you don't consume more fruit servings than vegetable servings. Almost the entire produce world is open for you to explore, but keep the following in mind.

It's thumbs down to the white potato. Though it's nutritious (it's filled with potassium), it sends your blood sugar levels soaring, which can increase cravings for more food.

Don't eat more than a few servings a week of starchy vegetables, such as pumpkin, winter squash, sweet potatoes, and yams. While these foods offer healthy vitamins and phytonutrients, they are also quite high in calories and carbohydrates.

Stay away from dried fruits. They are not as filling as raw fruits, are overly concentrated in calories and sugar, and are often treated with additives.

Choose whole fruits over fruit juices. Whole fruits offer more fiber and are more filling than juices.

Powerful Protein Foods

No matter how many calories you consume each day, you must eat three 8-ounce portions of protein foods. Protein sources include animal (meat, seafood, poultry), vegetable (beans, legumes, soy), and low-fat dairy (milk, yogurt, cottage cheese). You can divide your protein however you'd like throughout the day. Just be sure you eat some at each meal and that you reach your total of 24 ounces each day. Here are some hints.

Select a variety of proteins to consume throughout the day. That way you'll cover the nutritional spectrum and won't get bored.

Limit red meat servings to twice a week. This protein source tends to be higher in unhealthy saturated fat.

Avoid processed meats. They are usually high in fat and sodium nitrates.

(continued on page 126)

NOTES FOR THE CHEF FROM THE CHEF

Here are some hints to help when preparing the delicious recipes from *The Biggest Loser*.

Cooking Equipment

Though these recipes require no special equipment, we recommend that you consider purchasing the following items.

OLIVE OIL SPRAYER. There's a big difference between olive oil spray and olive oil cooking spray. The first is a sprayer that you fill with your favorite olive oil. The latter is a pre-filled, often aerosol spray that contains propellants and other ingredients. Using an olive oil sprayer gives you the option to lightly mist extra-virgin olive oil directly onto your food to improve the texture and flavor.

KITCHEN SCALE. Though we've tried to provide cup measurements for all ingredient amounts, we highly recommend that you invest in a kitchen scale if you truly want to live a healthy lifestyle. Often, when people are struggling with weight loss, the culprit is misjudged portion sizes.

DELI MEAT SLICER. Most deli meats are absolutely packed with sodium (up to 900 milligrams per 4-ounce serving). And the "lower-sodium" varieties aren't much better. If you're a big fan of deli sandwiches, you might want to consider investing in a meat slicer. Over time, you will save money by cooking turkey breasts and lean roasts instead of purchasing deli meats. Plus, you'll dramatically reduce your sodium intake.

Special Ingredients

Below are explanations of a few of the choices the experts on the show make that might not otherwise be clear; they will help you throughout this book and in your everyday healthier cooking.

LOW-CARB VERSUS LOW-FAT TORTILLAS. Though low-carb tortillas have more fiber and fewer carbs, they also tend to have much more sodium. If you're concerned about your sodium intake, be sure to check the labels. Also, low-fat varieties tend to have more whole grains and natural ingredients. If you're cooking the tortillas or making pizza crusts, it's essential that you opt for low-fat since low-carb tortillas don't crisp.

FRESH HERBS. Fresh herbs take time to chop, but they add loads of flavor without adding many calories. Fresh basil in a salad or fresh tarragon in an omelet can transform a boring meal into a gourmet feast—with no harm to your hips or your heart.

FRESH JUICES AND GARLIC. Though it's a bit more work to use fresh juices and fresh garlic, we can't even describe how much better they taste, compared to the bottled counterparts. For us, it's the difference between truly enjoying a dish and "stomaching it."

SODIUM AND SOUPS. Even though the Biggest Loser diet stresses a low-sodium intake, you'll notice that the soups in this book have higher amounts of sodium. Soups made with clear broths are vastly improved when using broth with lower sodium, as opposed to no-sodium broths. So when eating soup from this book (and many others), just be careful that your day hasn't been otherwise filled with sodium.

GROUND MEATS. If you have trouble finding extra-lean ground turkey, chicken, pork, veal, or even beef, don't despair. The butcher at most major grocery stores will grind meats for no charge. Not only will you know it's fresh, you may even save money over buying it pre-ground. One more thing to note: If you substitute ground turkey in dishes that traditionally call for beef, you may notice that the turkey has less moisture. Ground chicken also works well as a substitute.

LOW-FAT VERSUS FAT-FREE MAYONNAISE. Though the Biggest Loser diet recommends fat-free mayonnaise over low-fat, we've used low-fat throughout the book since we're willing to trade a few grams of fat and extra calories for better taste. If you like the taste of fat-free mayonnaise, or if you're really working to maximize your weight loss, just substitute fat-free mayonnaise.

LOW-FAT VERSUS FAT-FREE CHEESE. Again, we've chosen low-fat cheese over fat-free. As with mayo, it's your choice. One important note: When using low-fat or fat-free cheese, always shred it finely. You will need less to get some in every bite, and it will melt more like its full-fat counterpart.

BROWN RICE. We love short-grain brown rice. Though short-grain is less common, if you've only tried long-grain, it might be worth a visit to your local health food store. Short-grain has a nuttier flavor and a firmer texture that we prefer.

Wonderful Whole Grains

On the Biggest Loser diet, you'll be eating two 1-cup servings of whole grain foods each day. A whole grain is one that has undergone very little processing so that it retains its nutrients. Examples include barley, brown rice, bulgur, corn grits, couscous, cream of rice, cream of wheat, millet, oat bran, quinoa, rolled oats, whole wheat cereal, whole wheat pasta, and wild rice.

Try to avoid processed or refined carbohydrates, including most ready-to-eat breakfast cereals, which can be loaded with sugar. When choosing bread, look for "whole wheat" in the ingredient list. One bread serving is equal to 2 slices of whole-wheat bread (preferably "light"), 1 whole-wheat bun or roll, 1 whole-wheat flour tortilla, or 2 light Wasa crisp breads.

Extraordinary Extras

According to the Biggest Loser 4-3-2-1 Pyramid, you will be eating no more than 200 calories of extras a day. Now 200 calories sounds like a lot, but it's not as much food as you might think, so don't blow it on appetite-stimulating foods like white bread, white pasta, white potatoes, pastries, candy, and fruit snacks.

Instead, use your calorie budget wisely and spend it on healthy choices that will make your meals taste great. Extras can include oils such as olive, canola, flaxseed, and walnut; condiments such as mustard, horseradish, salsa, Tabasco, low-calorie ketchup, and low-calorie barbecue sauce; and splurges such as avocado, nuts and seeds, olives, and unsweetened pickles.

Eat reduced-fat, sugar-free, fat-free, and low-carb products sparingly, tempting as they might be. Same with artificial sweeteners, because you're aiming for meals that are as natural and nutritious as possible. Try using calorie-free extras such as garlic, herbs, spices, and vinegar to perk up your meals.

What Should You Drink?

The best and easiest beverage choice is water. You should drink 6 to 8 cups each day. If you find plain water boring, add herb sprigs, slices of cucumber, or citrus fruits.

Other beverages you can enjoy in moderation include no-calorie flavored water, coffee, tea (caffeinated or decaf), and herbal teas (hot or iced). If you're one of those dieters who chugs diet sodas, it's time to go cold turkey—well, almost. You should cut back to one or two a day. Non-diet soda is off-limits on the Biggest Loser diet; a 20-ounce bottle of soda can contain 17 teaspoons of sugar and 250 empty calories!

Alcohol, while limited, is not forbidden. You might choose to spend your 200 extra calories on a glass of wine, beer, or spirits. Wine, especially red, is the preferred alcohol choice because it has been proven to be heart-healthy and full of antioxidants. There are a few things to keep in mind about alcohol: It supplies calories but few nutrients; it might interfere with your body' ability to burn fat; and because it lowers inhibitions and stimulates appetite, it might cause you to engage in some unwise food choices.

WHAT IF YOU FEEL LIKE GIVING UP?

If you eat something you shouldn't, if you indulge on a special occasion, if you give yourself a break on vacation, it's normal. Don't beat yourself up, and whatever you do, don't give up. Get back on track as soon as you can.

The Biggest Loser
COOKBOOK

30 delicious recipes from the hit TV show

The recipes on the following pages show that healthy eating and successful weight loss don't mean giving up your favorite foods. Lose big with Steak Fajitas, Shrimp Quesadillas, Chocolate Cheesecakes, and more. Fight fat with these healthy recipes and become the Biggest Loser.

BREAKFASTS

Remember how your mom used to say, "Breakfast is the most important meal of the day"? Well, believe it or not, your mom was right, and her words of wisdom have been validated by the most recent studies in nutrition. These studies show that skipping breakfast can be a big contributor to weight gain.

So why is breakfast so important? First of all, you need it. Most of us use up more energy during the morning hours and therefore need the long-lasting fuel provided by a well-balanced breakfast. Even better, breakfast keeps you from getting hungry later in the day. If you eat a healthy meal in the morning, you will be less tempted to overeat in the afternoon—leading to better food choices throughout the day. In addition, breakfast kick-starts your brain, your body—and best of all, your metabolism—so that you think better, live better, and burn calories more efficiently.

Try carving out time for breakfast; you might really enjoy it. A relaxed morning meal can set the tone for a cheerful, productive day. And there's no better way to start off a day on the Biggest Loser diet than with Wild West Frittata, Family Favorite Breakfast Scramble, Subtly Strawberry Oatmeal, or our other breakfast greats.

WILD WEST FRITTATA

MAKES 4 SERVINGS

If you can't find an affordable ham steak in the cold meat section, you can always try the deli case. Just ask for one slice of extra-lean ham that is about ¼ inch thick. It's likely to be just about what you need.

¾ cup chopped sweet onion

½ cup chopped green bell pepper

4 ounces 97% or 98% lean ham steak, cut into ¼" cubes

Salt, to taste

Ground black pepper, to taste

2 cups egg substitute

2 ounces (1 cup) finely shredded light Swiss cheese

1. PREHEAT the broiler.

2. PLACE a medium broiler-safe nonstick skillet over medium heat. Lightly mist the skillet with the olive oil spray. Add the onion, bell pepper, and ham and cook for 5 to 7 minutes, or until the onion and pepper are softened but not browned. Season with salt and pepper (keep in mind that you will be adding ham and cheese, so you won't need much salt).

3. TURN the heat to medium-high and pour the egg substitute into the pan. Stir the veggies and ham in the eggs until they are evenly distributed and the eggs are slightly scrambled, 1 to 2 minutes. Reduce the heat to medium. Continue to cook, continuously sliding a spatula all around the sides of the frittata as far into the bottom as possible to loosen and gently lift the eggs slightly from the pan to prevent sticking, until the frittata is almost set but still runny on top, 4 to 6 minutes.

4. REMOVE the pan from the heat and sprinkle the cheese evenly over the top. Transfer the skillet to the oven and broil for 1 to 3 minutes, or until the cheese is melted and the egg is completely set. Cut the frittata into four equal wedges and serve.

NUTRITIONAL INFO PER SERVING: 142 calories, 22 g protein, 7 g carbohydrates, 2 g fat (2 g saturated), less than 1 g fiber, 621 mg sodium

FAMILY FAVORITE BREAKFAST SCRAMBLE

MAKES 4 SERVINGS

Scrambles are an easy way to start your day. Microwaving is a good way to scramble egg whites. Just be sure to continually push the cooked egg toward the middle of the bowl while microwaving, and they'll be perfectly fluffy and evenly cooked.

4 slices extra-lean turkey bacon, chopped

1 cup finely chopped sweet onion

2 teaspoons freshly minced garlic

16 large egg whites

3 cups loosely packed spinach leaves, stems removed

Salt, to taste

Ground black pepper, to taste

1. PLACE a large nonstick skillet over medium-high heat. Lightly mist the pan with the olive oil spray. Add the bacon, onion, and garlic and cook, stirring frequently, for 3 to 5 minutes, or until the onion is tender and the bacon is golden brown.

2. MEANWHILE, mist a large shallow microwave-safe bowl with the spray. Add the egg whites and cover the bowl with microwave-safe plastic wrap. Microwave on high for 1½ minutes. Uncover the bowl and, using a fork, push the cooked portions of the whites from the outside toward the middle of the bowl, letting the runny, uncooked parts run to the outer edge. Re-cover the bowl and microwave in 30-second intervals until the whites are just a bit runny on top. Uncover, then using a fork, stir the whites to break into large "scrambled" pieces. By the time you scramble and stir them, the residual heat should have cooked away the runniness. If they are still undercooked, re-cover and continue cooking in 10-second intervals until just done (be careful not to overcook).

3. ADD the scrambled egg whites and the spinach to the bacon mixture and stir well to wilt the spinach slightly and incorporate the egg whites. Season with salt and pepper. Divide the scramble among 4 plates and serve.

NUTRITIONAL INFO PER SERVING: 109 calories, 19 g protein, 6 g carbohydrates, less than 1 g fat (trace saturated), 1 g fiber, 381 mg sodium

SUBTLY STRAWBERRY OATMEAL

MAKES 1 SERVING

This simple oatmeal is given a touch of sweetness and a hint of strawberry using 100 percent fruit spread. Feel free to experiment with other flavors to add even more variety.

1 cup water

Pinch of salt

½ cup old-fashioned oats

½ teaspoon vanilla extract

1½ tablespoons 100% fruit strawberry preserves

1. **IN** a small saucepan, combine the water and salt and bring to a rapid boil over high heat. Add the oats and reduce the heat to medium. Cook, stirring occasionally, for 5 to 7 minutes, or until all the liquid is almost absorbed. Stir in the vanilla extract.

2. **COVER,** remove from the heat, and let sit for 5 minutes. Spoon into a serving bowl, stir in the preserves, and serve.

NUTRITIONAL INFO PER SERVING: 226 calories, 7 g protein, 42 g carbohydrates, 3 g fat (0 g saturated), 4 g fiber, 78 mg sodium

BOSTON-CREAM PEANUT-BUTTER BREAKFAST BANANA SPLIT

MAKES 1 SERVING

Who doesn't want a banana split . . . any time of the day? Here's one that's not only so decadent you'll forget you're eating healthy, and it's so fun, you're likely to feel like a kid again—a kid getting away with eating "junk food" for breakfast.

1 small ripe banana (about 6" long), peeled and halved lengthwise

1 tablespoon reduced-fat peanut butter

⅓ cup low-fat, artificially sweetened Boston cream pie–flavored yogurt

2 tablespoons crunchy high-fiber, low-sugar cereal (such as Grape-Nuts)

1. **PLACE** the banana halves in a small banana split dish or shallow bowl, with the cut sides facing inward. Spread the peanut butter evenly over the open banana.

2. **SPOON** the yogurt in the middle. Top with the cereal. Serve immediately.

NUTRITIONAL INFO PER SERVING: 294 calories, 8 g protein, 53 g carbohydrates, 7 g fat (2 g saturated), 5 g fiber, 241 mg sodium

BETTER BLUEBERRY PANCAKES

MAKES TWO 4-PANCAKE SERVINGS

If you're as big a fan of these pancakes as we are, rest assured that you can double, triple, and even quadruple this recipe with great success. In addition, the batter will keep in your refrigerator for up to 3 days.

½ cup reduced-fat buttermilk

½ cup whole grain oat flour

1 large egg white, lightly beaten

½ teaspoon baking soda

¼ teaspoon vanilla extract

¼ teaspoon salt

½ cup fresh or frozen (not thawed) blueberries

I Can't Believe It's Not Butter! spray

Sugar-free, low-calorie pancake syrup (optional)

100% fruit orange marmalade spread (optional)

1. **PREHEAT** the oven to 200°F.

2. **IN** a small bowl, combine the buttermilk, flour, egg white, baking soda, vanilla, and salt. Whisk just until blended. Stir in the blueberries. Let stand for 10 minutes.

3. **HEAT** a large nonstick skillet over medium heat until it is hot enough for a spritz of water to sizzle on it. With an oven mitt, briefly remove the pan from the heat to mist lightly with I Can't Believe It's Not Butter! cooking spray. Return the pan to the heat. Pour the batter in ⅛-cup dollops onto the skillet to form 3 or 4 pancakes. Cook for about 2 minutes, or until bubbles appear on the tops and the bottoms are golden brown. Flip. Cook for about 2 minutes, or until browned on the bottom.

4. **TRANSFER** to an oven-proof plate. Cover with aluminum foil. Place in the oven to keep warm. Repeat with cooking spray and the remaining batter to make 8 pancakes total.

5. **PLACE** 4 pancakes on each of 2 serving plates. Serve immediately with I Can't Believe It's Not Butter! spray, syrup, and/or fruit spread, if desired.

NUTRITIONAL INFO PER SERVING: 140 calories, 8 g protein, 20 g carbohydrates, 3 g fat (less than 1 g saturated), 3 g fiber, 687 mg sodium

HEARTY SNACKS

Forget about what diet gurus used to tell you about not snacking between meals. New research has shown that snacking is a great weight-loss strategy— as long as you're not snacking on unhealthy junk food. The recipes in this section are so delicious, you won't miss those fat-filled and sodium-loaded potato chips. There is enormous wisdom in eating frequently, which is why healthy snacking is one of the hallmarks of a successful dieter. It just makes sense that if you eat more often, you'll be hungry less often—safeguarding you from unhealthy temptations.

In addition, snacking helps you tame carb and sugar cravings. It aids in controlling blood sugar and insulin levels (insulin is a fat-forming hormone) and leads to lower body fat. Best of all, it keeps you from feeling deprived and it allows you to be flexible in the way you eat. On the Biggest Loser diet, you get to snack from one to three times a day, depending on your daily calorie goals.

Here are two of our favorite snacks.

CHAMP'S CHICKEN QUESADILLA

MAKES 1 SERVING

Not that long ago, many Americans had never heard of a quesadilla. Now many of us love them, but they're not the healthiest thing going. Fortunately, it's relatively easy to create a well-balanced healthy version!

¼ teaspoon chili powder

¼ teaspoon ground paprika

¼ teaspoon onion powder

Pinch of garlic powder

Pinch of ground cumin

Pinch of salt

2 ounces boneless, skinless chicken breast, trimmed of visible fat

1 whole wheat flour, 96% fat-free tortilla (8" diameter)

½ cup (1 ounce) finely shredded Cabot 75% Light Cheddar Cheese

1. **PREHEAT** the grill to high heat.

2. **IN** a small bowl, combine the chili powder, paprika, onion powder, garlic powder, cumin, and salt. Rub the mixture evenly over the chicken. Cover with plastic wrap and refrigerate for 10 minutes, for flavors to blend.

3. **PLACE** the chicken on the grill and lower the heat to medium. (If it is not possible to reduce the heat, sear the chicken quickly on both sides and then move away from direct heat.) Grill the chicken for 2 to 4 minutes per side, or until it is no longer pink and the juices run clear. Set aside for about 10 minutes. Chop the chicken coarsely.

4. **PREHEAT** a medium nonstick skillet over medium heat. With an oven mitt, briefly remove it from the heat to mist with olive oil spray. Lay the tortilla in the pan. Cook for 30 seconds. Flip the tortilla. Evenly scatter the cheese over half the tortilla. Top with the reserved chicken. With a spatula, fold the tortilla in half over the filling. Cook for 2 to 4 minutes, or until it starts to brown in spots. Flip and cook 2 to 4 minutes, or until the bottom starts to brown in spots and the cheese is melted. Slice into 4 wedges. Serve immediately.

NUTRITIONAL INFO PER SERVING: 242 calories, 26 g protein, 25 g carbohydrates, 5 g fat (2 g saturated), 3 g fiber, 454 mg sodium

GOURMET ROAST BEEF ROLL-UPS

MAKES 1 SERVING

These roll-ups are a great appetizer to take to a party. Not only will you look like a star for bringing such attractive, tasty food, if everything else is fried, you'll have something to munch on yourself. And you'll set yourself up to avoid unhealthy food without starving. Just be sure you use roast beef that's been shaved or is very thinly sliced; otherwise the tortillas will tear when you roll them. The chili garlic sauce is available in the international foods aisle of most major grocery stores with other Thai ingredients. If you can't find it, subbing in chili paste is okay, too.

1 tablespoon fat-free cream cheese

¼ to ½ teaspoon chili garlic sauce

1 whole wheat flour, 96% fat-free tortilla (8" diameter)

Scant ¼ cup roasted red bell pepper strips

¼ cup loosely packed chopped fresh basil leaves

¾ cup (3 ounces) lean, low-sodium deli roast beef

1. **IN** a small bowl, combine the cream cheese and chili garlic sauce to taste. Stir to mix well.

2. **PLACE** the tortilla on a cutting board. Spread the cheese mixture evenly over about two-thirds of the tortilla to the edges. Top the cream cheese mixture with the pepper strips, basil, and roast beef. Starting at the filled end, roll the tortilla tightly into a tube, being careful not to tear it.

3. **SPACE** 8 toothpicks evenly across it and poke them into the tube so they go through and touch the cutting board. With a sharp knife, cut between the picks to make 8 pieces. Take one piece and push the toothpick through so that the roll is evenly spaced in the center. Repeat with the remaining pieces. Arrange, spiral side up, on a serving plate. Serve immediately or cover with plastic wrap and refrigerate for up to 6 hours.

NUTRITIONAL INFO PER SERVING: 226 calories, 22 g protein, 30 g carbohydrates, 5 g fat (1 g saturated), 3 g fiber, 409 mg sodium

SANDWICHES AND SOUPS

The dishes in this section are rib-sticking, soul-satisfying, and downright comforting. After just one bite, you'll forget that you're eating healthy "diet" food. Soups and sandwiches lend themselves to healthful preparations without much change in flavor, texture, or pizzazz. Instead of a fatty burger with ground beef, try substituting ground turkey or chicken, like we did for the California Bacon Burger.

As you can tell from the recipes here, soups and sandwiches are really quite versatile. You can make them plain or fancy, you can serve them for lunch or dinner, and they're good in hot weather as well as cold. They also offer plenty of room for culinary creativity. Feel free to personalize these recipes by adding herbs, spices, or your favorite vegetables (as long as they're healthy, of course). These dishes are all bursting with flavors. We think you'll especially love the Indian Chicken Salad Pockets and Mom's New Beef Stew.

CALIFORNIA BACON BURGER

MAKES 1 SERVING

Bacon lovers, rejoice. This highly seasoned bacon burger is one of our favorites. True, it's a bit high in sodium, but worth every bite if your diet isn't otherwise full of sodium. You could alternate making it with extra-lean ground beef and turkey, and we encourage you to swap in and out ingredients to your taste . . . as long as you're sticking to lean ones. The tablespoon of egg substitute and bread crumbs help to achieve the texture of a fattier burger.

1 strip nitrate-free turkey bacon, cut in half

1 tablespoon egg substitute

1 tablespoon Ian's Whole Wheat Panko Breadcrumbs or finely crushed Wasa Light Rye Crispbread

¼ pound Jennie-O Turkey Store Extra-Lean Ground Turkey

1 tablespoon chopped fresh parsley leaves

1 teaspoon Worcestershire sauce

1 teaspoon minced fresh jalapeño chile pepper

¾ ounce very thinly sliced Cabot's 75% Light Cheddar Cheese

1 whole grain or whole wheat hamburger bun

1 tablespoon low-fat mayonnaise

3 tomato slices, or to taste

1 thin slice red onion, or to taste

1. **PLACE** a medium nonstick pan over medium-high heat. Place the bacon in the pan. Cook for 3 to 4 minutes per side, or until crisp. Transfer to a plate. Cover to keep warm.

2. **MEANWHILE,** in a small bowl, combine the egg substitute and bread crumbs or crushed crispbread. Add the turkey, parsley, Worcestershire sauce, and chile pepper. With clean hands or a fork, mix well. Shape into a patty that is about ½" wider than the bun.

3. **RETURN** the pan to medium-high heat until it is hot enough for a spritz of water to sizzle on it. With an oven mitt, briefly remove the pan from the heat to mist lightly with olive oil spray. Place the patty in the pan. Cook for about 2 minutes per side. Reduce the heat to medium. Cook for 2 minutes. Flip the patty. Cover it with cheese. Place the bun halves, cut side down, in the pan next to the patty. Cook for about 2 minutes, or until the turkey is no longer pink and the bun halves are toasted.

4. **PLACE** the bun bottom on a serving plate. Spread half of the mayonnaise over it. Top with the patty, bacon, tomato, and onion. Spread the remaining mayonnaise over the inside of the bun top. Flip onto the burger.

NUTRITIONAL INFO PER SERVING: 371 calories, 47 g protein, 27 g carbohydrates, 10 g fat (2 g saturated), 2 g fiber, 832 mg sodium

INDIAN CHICKEN SALAD POCKETS

MAKES 2 SERVINGS

Here's a simple trick: Mix low-fat mayonnaise with stronger flavors to give it the richness of a full-fat mayonnaise. Here, low-fat mayo combines with curry paste, which is found in the international foods aisle in most major grocery stores. Just be sure you don't go crazy with these pastes in other dishes because most are insanely full of fat and sodium. But they also have very strong flavor, so in a dish like this just ½ teaspoon does it.

1½ tablespoons low-fat mayonnaise

1 teaspoon lime juice, preferably fresh squeezed

½ teaspoon curry paste

¾ cup (4 ounces) chopped grilled chicken breast

1½ tablespoons seeded, chopped cucumber

1½ tablespoons chopped red onion

1 whole wheat pita (6½" diameter), cut in half

2 leaves green leaf lettuce

1. IN a medium bowl, combine the mayonnaise, lime juice, and curry paste. Whisk to blend. Add the chicken, cucumber, and onion. Mix well.

2. SPOON the mixture evenly into the pita halves. Add the lettuce. Serve immediately.

NUTRITIONAL INFO PER SERVING: 186 calories, 20 g protein, 16 g carbohydrates, 5 g fat (1 g saturated), 2 g fiber, 304 mg sodium

GRILLED CHEESE SANDWICH

MAKES 1 SERVING

Biggest Loser star Matt Kamont has always been a big fan of cheese. He says, "I love mac and cheese, grilled cheese, bacon-egg-and-cheese bagels . . . anything with cheese, really." When he got home from the ranch, he was really missing cheese. He was determined to find a way to eat a healthier version of his favorite foods so he didn't go crazy and binge. He went to the grocery store and picked up some light rye and light Cheddar, and now he can indulge in one of his all-time favorites.

2 slices light rye bread

1½ ounces paper-thin slices Cabot 75% Light Cheddar Cheese

I Can't Believe It's Not Butter! spray

1. PLACE one slice of bread on a serving plate. Top evenly with the cheese and the remaining slice of bread.

2. PREHEAT a small nonstick pan over medium heat until it is hot enough for a spritz of water to sizzle on it. With an oven mitt, briefly remove the pan from the heat to mist lightly with I Can't Believe It's Not Butter! spray. Place the sandwich in the pan. Cook for 3 to 4 minutes, or until the bread is lightly browned. Carefully flip the sand-wich. Cook for 3 to 4 minutes, or until the cheese is completely melted. Serve immediately.

NUTRITIONAL INFO PER SERVING: 189 calories, 18 g protein, 19 g carbohydrates, 6 g fat (2 g saturated), 6 g fiber, 490 mg sodium

BLACK BEAN SOUP

If you don't have an immersion blender, don't worry. You can still make this recipe. Just bring the mixture to a simmer for a minute, then transfer to a traditional blender or food processor and puree. Be sure to put the lid on tight and drape a towel over the top of the blender, then hold to keep in place as you blend. Once it's smooth, you can pour it back into the saucepan and continue.

2 (15-ounce) cans 50% less sodium black beans, drained

1 (14.5-ounce) can diced tomatoes in juice

2 cups water

¾ cup minced celery

¾ cup minced onion

2 teaspoons finely chopped seeded jalapeño chile pepper (wear plastic gloves when handling)

1 teaspoon freshly minced garlic

1 teaspoon ground cumin

Ground black pepper

Red-pepper flakes

1. IN a large nonstick saucepan, combine three-fourths of the black beans, one-half of the tomatoes, and the water, and bring to a simmer over medium heat. With an immersion blender, puree until mostly smooth. (Note: When using an immersion blender, make sure not to scratch the bottom of your nonstick pan.) Add the remaining black beans and tomatoes, along with the celery, onion, jalapeño, garlic, and cumin. Season with black pepper and red-pepper flakes. Cover the pot, leaving the lid slightly ajar for steam to escape, and reduce the heat to low.

2. SIMMER for 20 to 25 minutes longer, or until the vegetables are tender. Divide the soup evenly among 6 soup bowls and serve.

NUTRITIONAL INFO PER SERVING: 84 calories, 5 g protein, 19 g carbohydrates, 0.1 g fat (0 g saturated fat), 6 g fiber, 387 mg sodium

MOM'S NEW BEEF STEW

MAKES FOUR 2¼-CUP SERVINGS

Don't worry, this stew isn't only for moms, but it's sure to taste as good as the one you grew up with. This is a great recipe for a Sunday afternoon while you're home doing the laundry. You'll have a great dinner and plenty of leftovers, which are just as good, if not better. Somewhere between 1½ and 2 hours of simmering, the meat will become extremely tender. If it is still tough, simmer it a bit longer.

1 tablespoon whole grain oat flour

⅛ teaspoon garlic powder

⅛ teaspoon salt, plus more to taste

Pinch of ground black pepper, plus more to taste

1 pound top round steak, cut into 1" cubes

2 teaspoons extra-virgin olive oil

8 ounces button mushrooms, each halved

1 onion, cut into bite-size pieces

1 tablespoon minced garlic

1 teaspoon dried thyme

2 cans (14 ounces each) lower-sodium, fat-free beef broth

2 large carrots, peeled and cut into bite-size pieces

1 pound sweet potatoes, peeled and cut into 1" cubes

1. IN a medium resealable plastic bag, combine the flour, garlic powder, salt, and pepper. Add the beef and shake the bag until all the cubes are coated. Refrigerate for at least 15 minutes.

2. SET a large nonstick soup pot over medium-high heat until it is hot enough for a spritz of water to sizzle on it. Add the oil. Add the reserved beef cubes to the pot in a single layer. Cook for about 1 minute per side, or until browned. Reduce the heat to medium. Add the mushrooms, onion, garlic, and thyme. Cook, stirring occasionally with a wooden spoon and scraping any browned bits from the pan bottom, for about 10 minutes, or until the onion is tender.

3. ADD the broth and carrots. Increase the heat to high. When the broth comes to a boil, reduce the heat to low so the mixture simmers gently. Cover and cook for 45 minutes.

4. ADD the potatoes. Cook for 45 minutes, or until the beef is fork-tender. Season with additional salt and pepper. Serve immediately.

NUTRITIONAL INFO PER SERVING: 275 calories, 31 g protein, 29 g carbohydrates, 6 g fat (2 g saturated), 6 g fiber, 583 mg sodium

SALADS

Salads are nutritious and delicious, but best of all, they're supremely satisfying. Why? Because they take a long time to eat, they're crunchy, and they're filling. You can indulge in a healthy salad with every meal on the Biggest Loser diet—in fact, you should. According to the Biggest Loser diet plan, you should eat a minimum of 4 servings of fruits and vegetables daily. But when we say *minimum*, that means that you can eat more.

Let your creativity run wild when it comes to salads (or just turn to one of the salad recipes in this section). It's amazing how much beautiful produce is available at your local supermarket; your neighborhood farmers' market will have even more! There are so many fantastic greens out there that there's just no excuse for a boring salad made from plain old iceberg. For crunch, you can add peppers, cucumber, or celery. For color and flavor, try tomatoes or red onions; for taste and bulk try a blanched green vegetable. And don't forget about sliced mushrooms or bean sprouts. They add lots of volume and texture with hardly any calories.

Even though you'll need to avoid high-fat salad dressings and add-ons, there are other ways to liven up your greens. Try dressing your salads with "good" fats, reduced-fat or fat-free salad dressings, a bit of avocado, or some nuts or seeds. And, of course, you can always add herbs, spices, garlic, lemon or lime juice, and vinegar to your salads with no extra calorie charge!

GREEK SALAD WITH GRILLED CHICKEN

MAKES 4 SERVINGS

This delicious salad includes an unusual vinaigrette with a zesty yellow mustard taste. If you haven't had a lot of fat in your day, you can throw in a few Greek olives to make the salad even more heavenly. But either way, if you love yellow mustard, you'll love this salad.

12 cups chopped fresh spinach leaves

3 cups chopped tomatoes

2 cups chopped cucumber

3 ounces crumbled reduced-fat feta cheese

Greek vinaigrette (recipe below)

1 pound lean grilled chicken breast, sliced

1. **IN** a large glass or plastic bowl, combine the spinach, tomatoes, cucumber, and feta. Pour the vinaigrette over the mixture and toss.

2. **DIVIDE** the salad among 4 dinner plates or large salad bowls. Top each with one-fourth of the chicken (about 4 ounces) and serve.

NUTRITIONAL INFO PER SERVING: 268 calories, 35 g protein, 14 g carbohydrates, 9 g fat (3 g saturated), 4 g fiber, 637 mg sodium

GREEK VINAIGRETTE

MAKES 4 SERVINGS

3 tablespoons yellow mustard

2 tablespoons apple cider vinegar

1 tablespoon fat-free plain yogurt

1½ teaspoons honey

1 tablespoon extra-virgin olive oil

2 tablespoons minced onion

1 teaspoon freshly minced garlic

Pinch of salt

Ground black pepper

1. **IN** a medium resealable plastic container, whisk together the mustard, vinegar, yogurt, and honey. Slowly whisk in the oil. Stir in the onion and garlic, then season with salt and pepper.

2. **SERVE** immediately or store in the refrigerator for up to 5 days.

NUTRITIONAL INFO PER SERVING: 62 calories, 1 g protein, 6 g carbohydrates, 4 g fat (.5 g saturated fat), less than 1 g fiber, 203 mg sodium

SPINACH SALAD WITH FETA AND MANDARIN ORANGES

MAKES 4 SERVINGS

The sweetness of the oranges in this salad and the saltiness of the feta, coupled with lean protein and fresh spinach, help keep cravings satisfied. Be sure to always dry raw veggies well. That's how to achieve restaurant-quality salads!

14 cups loosely packed spinach leaves, stems removed

1 can (10½-ounce) unsweetened mandarin oranges in juice, drained (about 1 cup)

1½ ounces finely crumbled reduced-fat feta cheese

½ cup red onion slivers

6 tablespoons light balsamic vinaigrette

1 pound lean grilled chicken breast, cut into strips

1. **IN** a large salad bowl, combine the spinach, oranges, feta, and onion. Pour the vinaigrette over the mixture and toss.

2. **DIVIDE** the salad among 4 dinner plates or large salad bowls. Top each with one-fourth of the chicken (about 4 ounces) and serve.

NUTRITIONAL INFO PER SERVING: 240 calories, 31 g protein, 17 g carbohydrates, 6 g fat (2 g saturated), 5 g fiber, 469 mg sodium

DELI CHOPPED SALAD

By chopping the ingredients for this salad finely, the flavors mix, so you don't need to use exorbitant amounts of dressing to get a flavor explosion with every bite. If you don't plan on enjoying this main-dish salad immediately, don't add the dressing until just before serving. And be sure to remove the seeds from the tomato, which can also make your salad soggy over time.

3 cups finely chopped romaine lettuce leaves

½ cup (2 ounces) diced lean, low-sodium deli-style turkey

⅓ cup (1½ ounces) diced lean, low-sodium deli-style roast beef

⅓ cup (1½ ounces) diced low-fat mozzarella cheese

½ cup finely chopped, seeded tomato

¼ cup loosely packed fresh basil leaves, finely chopped

3 tablespoons finely chopped red onion

2 tablespoons low-fat Italian salad dressing

Red-pepper flakes, to taste (optional)

1. IN a large serving bowl, combine the lettuce, turkey, beef, cheese, tomato, basil, onion, and dressing. Toss to coat the ingredients with the dressing.

2. SEASON with pepper flakes, if desired. Serve immediately.

NUTRITIONAL INFO PER SERVING: 289 calories, 36 g protein, 18 g carbohydrates, 10 g fat (3 g saturated), 7 g fiber, 632 mg sodium

MAIN COURSES

After a long day on the job, at school, or taking care of the kids, it's hard to find the time or energy to whip up dinner—especially one that's healthy and well-balanced. It's no wonder that so many of us drive through the local fast food joint, pick up prepared food from the neighborhood market, call up for pizza or Chinese food, or pop something frozen in the microwave. When you're exhausted and in a hurry, it's natural to want to take the path of least resistance.

But as hard as it is to believe, there really is an alternative—like the recipes in this section. Many are quick and easy, and they're all healthy and guaranteed to please the entire family—including children. Who wouldn't love dishes like Rosemary-Grilled London Broil or Winning "Fried" Chicken?

Cooking requires a little bit of advance planning, but you'll find that taking a bit of time to organize and shop will pay off—in dollars saved and pounds lost! Try doing prep work in the morning before you leave the house so that you can hit the ground running when you get home.

Nothing satisfies like a home-cooked meal that requires minimum effort. Wouldn't you love to come home to something like Grilled Turkey Cutlets with Salsa?

ENCHILADA CHICKEN

MAKES 4 SERVINGS

Many of the Biggest Losers cite Enchilada Chicken as one of their favorite cheat foods. There's no cheating involved with this healthy version!

4 small (¼ pound) trimmed boneless, skinless chicken breasts, trimmed of all visible fat

2 teaspoons salt-free Mexican or Southwest seasoning (such as Mrs. Dash Southwest Chipotle)

Olive oil spray

4 tablespoons medium, mild, or hot enchilada sauce

1 cup (2 ounces) finely shredded Cabot's 75% Light Cheddar Cheese

2 tablespoons finely chopped fresh cilantro

1. PREHEAT the oven to 350°F.

2. SEASON each chicken breast evenly on all sides with the seasoning.

3. PLACE a large ovenproof nonstick skillet over high heat. When hot, lightly mist with the olive oil spray and add the chicken. Cook, turning once, for 1 to 2 minutes per side, or just until the chicken is golden brown on the outsides.

4. REMOVE the pan from the heat and top each chicken breast with 1 tablespoon of the enchilada sauce, followed by one-fourth of the cheese and one-fourth of the cilantro.

5. TRANSFER the skillet to the oven and bake for 4 to 6 minutes, or until the chicken is no longer pink inside and the cheese is melted.

NUTRITIONAL INFO PER SERVING: 162 calories, 31 g protein, 1 g carbohydrates, 3 g fat (1 g saturated), trace fiber, 230 mg sodium

GRILLED CHICKEN PARMESAN

MAKES 4 SERVINGS

Serve this simple dish with a side of whole wheat pasta and a large green salad. It's sure to be a hit!

4 small (¼ pound) boneless, skinless chicken breasts, trimmed of all visible fat

Olive oil in a sprayer (not store-bought spray that contains propellant)

Salt, to taste

Ground black pepper, to taste

½ cup low-fat, low-sodium, low-sugar marinara sauce, or more to taste

6 tablespoons finely shredded low-fat mozzarella cheese

2 tablespoons grated reduced-fat Parmesan cheese

1. PREHEAT the oven to 350°F. Preheat a grill to high heat.

2. LIGHTLY mist both sides of the chicken with olive oil and season with salt and pepper. Grill the chicken, turning once, for 3 to 5 minutes per side, or until it is no longer pink inside and juices run clear. Transfer to a baking dish.

3. HEAT the sauce on low in the microwave until warm. Top each breast with 2 tablespoons marinara sauce, followed by 1½ tablespoons mozzarella, and ½ tablespoon Parmesan.

4. BAKE the chicken for 3 to 5 minutes, or just until the cheese is melted.

NUTRITIONAL INFO PER SERVING: 169 calories, 29 g protein, 5 g carbohydrates, 3 g fat (less than 1 g saturated), 1 g fiber, 210 mg sodium

WINNING "FRIED" CHICKEN

This "fried" chicken is incredibly versatile. It's great as is, and it's also an awesome base for chicken Parmesan. Simply add a bit of marinara sauce and some low-fat mozzarella cheese. You could also chop it up to top a salad that is drizzled with a bit of wing sauce (just be careful of the sodium on that one). Oh, and in case you are wondering, panko is Japanese bread crumbs that are super crispy. They are ideal for faux fried foods because you don't need to add oil to achieve perfectly crisp breading. If you can't find panko, a second choice is crushed-up Wasa crispbread.

3 tablespoons fat-free plain yogurt

4 large fresh basil leaves, chopped

1 teaspoon chopped fresh oregano leaves

1 teaspoon chopped fresh thyme leaves

¼ teaspoon garlic powder

Pinch of salt

Pinch of ground black pepper

4 tablespoons Ian's Whole Wheat Panko Breadcrumbs or finely crushed Wasa Light Rye Crispbread

2 small (¼-pound) boneless, skinless chicken breasts, trimmed of visible fat

Mustard or low-fat, low-sodium marinara sauce, to taste (optional)

1. PREHEAT the oven to 400°F. Lightly mist a small nonstick baking sheet with olive oil spray.

2. IN a medium shallow bowl, combine the yogurt, basil, oregano, thyme, garlic powder, salt, and pepper. Stir to mix well.

3. PLACE 2 tablespoons of the bread crumbs or crushed crispbread in another medium shallow bowl. Set next to the yogurt mixture. Dip 1 chicken breast into the yogurt mixture to coat. Transfer to the crumbs to coat evenly. Place on the prepared baking sheet. Add the remaining 2 tablespoons crumbs to the bowl. Repeat the procedure with the second breast. Place on the baking sheet, not touching the other breast.

4. BAKE for 10 minutes. Flip the chicken and bake for 8 to 10 minutes, or until no longer pink. Serve immediately with mustard or marinara sauce on the side, if desired.

NUTRITIONAL INFO PER SERVING: 173 calories, 29 g protein, 9 g carbohydrates, 2 g fat (less than 1 g saturated), 1 g fiber, 171 mg sodium

GRILLED TURKEY CUTLETS WITH SALSA

MAKES 4 SERVINGS

Grilling turkey cutlets makes them cook so quickly and much more evenly than larger cuts of turkey. This dish can be made with numerous varieties of salsa, so you're not likely to tire of it.

1 teaspoon extra-virgin olive oil

1 pound boneless, skinless turkey cutlets

⅛ to ¼ teaspoon seasoned salt, to taste

½ teaspoon salt-free, extra spicy seasoning (such as Mrs. Dash Extra Spicy)

6 tablespoons fresh salsa (refrigerated, not jarred), any variety

1. PREHEAT the grill to high heat.

2. RUB the oil all over the cutlets and season evenly with the seasoned salt and seasoning. Grill about 1 minute per side, or until no longer pink inside. Transfer the cutlets to a platter, top with the salsa, and serve.

NUTRITIONAL INFO PER SERVING: 134 calories, 28 g protein, 2 g carbohydrates, 2 g fat (trace saturated), 0 g fiber, 155 mg sodium

BBQ BACON MEAT LOAF

MAKES 4 SERVINGS

Bread crumbs are traditionally used in meat loaf and meatballs to add moisture to the finished dish and sometimes to add bulk to stretch the meat for your dollar. This recipe uses oatmeal instead because it will do the trick to create moist and delicious dishes while adding fiber, instead of just a bunch of white flour.

1 cup chopped red onion

4 slices extra-lean turkey bacon, chopped

⅔ cup old-fashioned oats

½ cup fat-free milk

1 pound extra-lean ground chicken breast

2 large egg whites, lightly beaten

1 clove fresh garlic, minced

1 teaspoon Worcestershire sauce

⅛ teaspoon salt

⅓ cup barbecue sauce (7 grams carbohydrates or less per 2 tablespoons)

1. **PREHEAT** the oven to 350°F. Lightly mist a 9" x 5" x 3" nonstick loaf pan with the olive oil spray.

2. **PLACE** a medium nonstick skillet over medium-high heat. Lightly mist the pan with spray and add the onion and bacon. Cook, stirring, for 6 to 8 minutes, or until the onion is tender and just barely starting to brown and the bacon is crisped. Remove the pan from the heat and allow the mixture to cool.

3. **COMBINE** the oats and milk in a medium mixing bowl and stir to mix. Let the mixture stand for 3 minutes, or until the oats begin to soften. Add the cooled onion and bacon mixture, the chicken, egg whites, garlic, Worcestershire sauce, and salt. With a fork or clean hands, mix the ingredients until well combined.

4. **TRANSFER** the mixture to the prepared pan and spread so the top is flat. Spread the barbecue sauce evenly over the top. Bake for 35 to 40 minutes, or until the chicken is completely cooked through and no longer pink. Let the loaf sit for 10 minutes before cutting into 8 slices to serve.

NUTRITIONAL INFO PER SERVING: 258 calories, 35 g protein, 20 g carbohydrates, 3 g fat (trace saturated), 2 g fiber, 529 mg sodium

INDIVIDUAL SAUSAGE-RIGATONI BAKE

MAKES 1 SERVING

Many people trying to lose weight try to give up sausage. But you can season the leanest cut of pork just like sweet Italian sausage. Simple!

SAUSAGE

3 ounces extra-lean ground pork

½ teaspoon fennel seeds

½ teaspoon dried parsley

¼ teaspoon red-pepper flakes

¼ teaspoon Italian seasoning

⅛ teaspoon garlic powder

Pinch of salt

RIGATONI AND SAUCE

¾ cup whole wheat rigatoni

⅔ cup thin, 1"-long red or yellow bell pepper strips

1 cup canned crushed tomatoes

1 tablespoon no-salt-added tomato paste

1 tablespoon water

1½ teaspoons dried oregano

½ teaspoon honey

¼ teaspoon garlic powder

2 teaspoons grated reduced-fat Parmesan cheese

1. **PREHEAT** the oven to 400°F.

2. **COMBINE** the pork, fennel seeds, parsley, pepper flakes, Italian seasoning, garlic powder, and salt. With clean hands or a fork, mix well.

3. **PLACE** a medium nonstick skillet over medium-high heat until it is hot enough for a spritz of water to sizzle on it. With an oven mitt, briefly remove the pan from the heat to lightly mist with olive oil spray.

4. **ADD** the sausage to the pan. Cook, breaking it into large chunks with a wooden spoon, for 3 to 5 minutes, or until no longer pink. Remove from the pan and cover to keep warm.

5. **LIGHTLY MIST** a 2- to 3-cup baking dish with olive oil spray. Set aside.

6. **COOK** the pasta according to package directions. Drain and set aside.

7. **MEANWHILE,** return the skillet to the heat, add the pepper strips, and cook 3 to 5 minutes until tender. Add the reserved sausage. Add the tomatoes, tomato paste, water, oregano, honey, and garlic powder. Stir to mix well. Add the reserved pasta. Transfer to the prepared baking dish. Sprinkle evenly with the cheese. Cover with aluminum foil.

8. **BAKE** for 10 minutes. Remove foil. Bake for 5 minutes, or until heated and the top is brown. Let stand for 5 minutes before serving.

NUTRITIONAL INFO PER SERVING: 427 calories, 30 g protein, 66 g carbohydrates, 7 g fat (1 g saturated), 12 g fiber, 629 mg sodium

STEAK FAJITAS

MAKES 4 SERVINGS

To get hot, sizzling, restaurant-style fajitas, you want to be sure to cook the steak strips in a single layer over high heat. That way, each strip of meat sears and browns on the outside, while the inside stays tender and juicy. Cooking the strips will be a very quick process (like cooking steak in a wok for a stir-fry), so make sure you watch as they cook and that you remove the meat from the pan as soon as it's done.

8 fajita-sized (about 6") low-carb, whole wheat flour tortillas

1½ teaspoons salt-free Southwest or Mexican seasoning

1 (1-pound) London broil, cut against the grain into strips

Salt, to taste

2 large green bell peppers, cut into strips

1 medium onion, cut into strips

1 tablespoon freshly minced garlic

¼ cup fat-free sour cream

½ cup fresh salsa or pico de gallo (refrigerated, not jarred), drained if watery

4 teaspoons minced seeded jalapeño chile pepper (Wear plastic gloves when handling.)

1. **PREHEAT** the oven to 400°F.

2. **STACK** the tortillas on a large sheet of foil and roll it into a tube to enclose the tortillas. Seal the ends. Heat the tortillas in the oven about 5 minutes, or until warm.

3. **SPRINKLE** the seasoning evenly over the steak strips and season with salt. Toss the meat well. Place a large nonstick skillet over medium-high heat. When hot, lightly mist with the olive oil spray. Add the bell peppers and cook, stirring, until beginning to soften, 3 to 5 minutes. Add the onion and garlic and cook, stirring, until tender and lightly browned, about 5 minutes. Transfer the vegetables to a bowl and cover to keep warm. Return the skillet to high heat. When hot, respray the pan. In batches if necessary, add the steak strips in a single layer. Cook, stirring occasionally, until the meat is lightly browned on the outsides and slightly pink inside, 1 to 2 minutes. Add the sautéed vegetables and toss with the meat until warm.

4. **UNROLL** the tortillas. Place 2 of them side by side on each of 4 large dinner plates. Divide the steak mixture among the tortillas, and top with the sour cream and salsa or pico de gallo. Sprinkle jalapeño over the fajitas and serve.

NUTRITIONAL INFO PER SERVING: 371 calories, 32 g protein, 52 g carbohydrates, 8 g fat (3 g saturated), 6 g fiber, 814 mg sodium

ROSEMARY-GRILLED LONDON BROIL

MAKES SIX 4-OUNCE SERVINGS

This roast is so simple, it only takes about 15 minutes from start to finish. You'll have a delicious dinner and leftovers that are a great alternative to deli meats that are often full of sodium and fillers. Just be sure to slice it extremely thin (almost shaved) by hand on a meat slicer for sandwiches or cut it into small cubes (½ inch is great) to throw into salads. Bigger pieces or thicker slices might seem tough after it's been chilled.

1 tablespoon minced garlic

1½ teaspoons dried rosemary

½ teaspoon extra-virgin olive oil

¼ teaspoon salt

¼ teaspoon ground black pepper

2 pounds beef London broil, trimmed of visible fat

1. **PREHEAT** the grill to high heat.

2. **IN** a small dish, combine the garlic, rosemary, oil, salt, and pepper. Rub the garlic mixture evenly over the roast. Let the beef stand 5 minutes.

3. **GRILL** the beef for 5 to 6 minutes per side, or until desired doneness. (A thermometer inserted in the center registers 145°F for medium-rare/160°F for medium/165°F for well done.) Tent it with foil and let stand for 10 minutes. Cut into thin slices against the grain of the meat. Serve immediately.

NUTRITIONAL INFO PER SERVING: 175 calories, 33 g protein, 5 g carbohydrates, 5 g fat (2 g saturated), trace fiber, 173 mg sodium

SWEET-AND-SPICY PORK TENDERLOIN

MAKES 4 SERVINGS

When it's cooked right, pork tenderloin is as tender as can be.

½ teaspoon ground cumin

½ teaspoon ground cinnamon

½ teaspoon salt

¼ teaspoon ground black pepper

¼ teaspoon ground allspice

⅛ teaspoon garlic powder

⅛ teaspoon ground chipotle chile pepper

1 pork tenderloin (1¼ pounds), trimmed of visible fat

1 teaspoon extra-virgin olive oil

2 tablespoons honey

1 tablespoon minced garlic

1½ teaspoons hot-pepper sauce

1. PREHEAT the oven to 350°F. Lightly mist a small roasting pan or ovenproof skillet with olive oil spray. Set aside.

2. IN a small bowl, combine the cumin, cinnamon, salt, black pepper, allspice, garlic powder, and chipotle pepper. Rub the pork evenly with the olive oil. Then rub evenly with the spice mixture until coated. Cover loosely with plastic wrap. Refrigerate for 15 minutes.

3. MEANWHILE, in a small bowl, combine the honey, garlic, and hot-pepper sauce. Whisk to mix. Set aside.

4. SET a large nonstick skillet over medium-high heat until it is hot enough for a spritz of water to sizzle on it. With an oven mitt, briefly remove the pan from the heat to lightly mist with olive oil spray. Place the pork in the pan. Cook for 1 minute per side, or until browned on all sides. Transfer to the prepared pan. With a basting brush, evenly coat the pork with the reserved honey mixture.

5. ROAST the tenderloin in the oven for 16 to 18 minutes, or until a thermometer inserted in the center reaches 160°F and the juices run clear. Remove from the oven. Cover the pork loosely with aluminum foil. Let stand for 10 minutes. Transfer the pork to a cutting board. Holding a knife at a 45° angle, cut into thin slices. Serve immediately.

NUTRITIONAL INFO PER SERVING: 221 calories, 30 g protein, 10 g carbohydrates, 6 g fat (2 g saturated), less than 1 g fiber, 375 mg sodium

SHRIMP QUESADILLAS

MAKES 1 SERVING

This quesadilla is perfect for people who enjoy mild flavors. If you have bolder tastes, feel free to add fresh cilantro or some salt-free Mexican seasoning. This recipe calls for bay shrimp to keep the cost low, but if larger shrimp are on sale, swap them in, though you'll need to cook the shrimp a bit longer and then chop them into smaller pieces.

2 teaspoons cocktail sauce

2 teaspoons fat-free sour cream

3 ounces cooked peeled bay shrimp (about ½ cup), drained

1 low-fat, low-carb, multigrain or whole wheat flour tortilla (7½" diameter)

¾ ounce (about ⅓ cup) finely shredded Cabot's 75% Light Cheddar Cheese or other low-fat Cheddar

1. IN a small bowl, mix the cocktail sauce and sour cream until thoroughly combined.

2. PLACE a small nonstick skillet over high heat. When hot, spray with the olive oil spray. Add the shrimp and cook for 1 to 2 minutes just to remove any excess moisture and heat the shrimp through.

3. PLACE a nonstick skillet large enough for the tortilla to lie flat in over medium-high heat and add the tortilla. Sprinkle about half of the cheese evenly over half of the tortilla. Top with the shrimp, followed by the remaining cheese. Fold the bare half over the filled half. Cook for about 2 minutes, or until the cheese begins to melt and the tortilla is lightly browned in spots. Carefully turn over and cook until the cheese is completely melted, 1 to 2 minutes longer.

4. TRANSFER the quesadilla to a serving plate and cut into 4 wedges. Serve immediately with the cocktail sauce mixture for dipping or dollop it on the quesadilla.

NUTRITIONAL INFO PER SERVING: 285 calories, 25 g protein, 17 g carbohydrates, 5 g fat (1 g saturated), 8 g fiber, 638 mg sodium

BLACKENED CATFISH

If you're looking for a fresh dinner in a flash, you can't possibly go wrong with this dish. It takes only about 15 minutes to make, but you'd never guess from the taste. You can buy catfish that has been flash frozen and keep it in your freezer. The night before or the morning of the day you plan to serve it, move it to the fridge. By the time dinner hits, it'll be defrosted and ready to go. If you forget to defrost it, run it under cold (not hot) water for about 10 minutes, and then lightly squeeze the moisture from it.

1 small (¼-pound) catfish fillet

¼ teaspoon blackened seasoning, or more to taste

½ teaspoon grated reduced-fat Parmesan cheese

1. PREHEAT the oven to 450°F. Lightly mist a small nonstick baking sheet with olive oil spray. Place the catfish, smooth-side down, on the sheet. Sprinkle on the blackened seasoning and cheese.

2. BAKE for 10 to 12 minutes, or until the catfish flakes easily with a fork. Serve immediately.

NUTRITIONAL INFO PER SERVING: 110 calories, 19 g protein, 0 g carbohydrates, 3 g fat (less than 1 g saturated), 0 g fiber, 165 mg sodium

SWEET SNACKS

There's no denying that most of us have a fearsome sweet tooth. It's one of the hardest things to reckon with when trying to lose weight. But we've got some good news for you: The recipes in this section will satisfy your sweet tooth, whether you're enjoying the treats as midday snacks or as desserts.

We all know that traditional desserts and sweet snacks are fattening, but it's not just the calorie count in a chocolate doughnut that makes it hard to reach your weight-loss goals. Most sweets are filled with white sugar and white flour, which are appetite stimulators. These ingredients have been stripped of their fiber and, when digested, the sugar and refined starch cause your blood sugar to skyrocket. In response, your body overreacts, pumping out so much insulin that your blood sugar plummets. When your blood sugar is low, you feel tired, cranky, hungry, and in need of a quick food fix, often in the form of something sweet. And *voila*—there's the vicious circle that wreaks havoc on your diet.

The key, of course, is to avoid appetite-stimulating foods and reach for natural, wholesome items instead. But that doesn't mean that the sweet snacks in this chapter will taste like "health food." What's not to love about Peanut Butter–Oatmeal Cookies, Chocolate-Kahlúa Mousse Parfaits, and Iced Buffed Mocha?

PEANUT BUTTER–OATMEAL COOKIES

MAKES TWO 2-COOKIE SERVINGS

Peanut butter cookies in a healthy cookbook? Yep! These no-bake cookies are made with dates, and the cool part is that the sugars found in dates are natural sugars that your body can easily process. Though you still don't want to eat a whole container of the cookies, when enjoyed in moderation they definitely curb a sweet tooth and a peanut butter craving all at once.

12 pitted dates

⅓ cup old-fashioned oats

1 tablespoon reduced-fat peanut butter

1. PLACE the dates in the bowl of a mini–food processor fitted with the chopping blade. Process until the dates are very finely chopped and stick together.

2. WITH a spatula, transfer to a small mixing bowl. Add the oats and peanut butter. Using an electric mixer fitted with beaters or your hands, mix well.

3. DIVIDE the mixture into 4 equal amounts. Shape each into a ball. Place one ball between two sheets of waxed paper. Flatten the ball to a 3"-diameter cookie. Repeat with each ball. Serve immediately or stack between sheets of waxed paper in an airtight plastic container. Refrigerate for up to 5 days.

NUTRITIONAL INFO PER SERVING: 221 calories, 5 g protein, 45 g carbohydrates, 4 g fat (less than 1 g saturated), 5 g fiber, 63 mg sodium

ONE-SERVING CHOCOLATE CHEESECAKES

MAKES 4 SERVINGS

Making desserts in single-serving sizes helps with portion control. When faced with an entire cheesecake, it's easy to feel justified in having "just another sliver." Try not to "whip" the cheesecake mixture on too high of a speed, or the finished cakes will get cracks in the top. Be sure to beat it on medium speed until just combined.

I Can't Believe It's Not Butter! spray

¼ cup crunchy high-fiber, low-sugar cereal (such as Grape-Nuts), finely crushed into crumbs

½ cup fat-free cream cheese, at room temperature

2 tablespoons honey

1 large egg white

¼ cup fat-free, artificially sweetened vanilla yogurt

¼ teaspoon vanilla extract

¼ cup cocoa powder, plus more for garnish

4 tablespoons aerosol fat-free whipped topping

1. **PREHEAT** the oven to 350°F.

2. **LIGHTLY** mist four 3"-wide ovenproof bowls or ramekins with I Can't Believe It's Not Butter! spray. Divide the crumbs among them, spreading in an even layer on the bottoms. Set aside.

3. **IN** a small mixing bowl, with an electric mixer fitted with beaters, beat the cream cheese and honey on medium speed until smooth. Add the egg white, yogurt, and vanilla extract. Beat on medium speed just until smooth. On the lowest speed possible, mix in the cocoa. Spoon the mixture into the prepared bowls or ramekins.

4. **BAKE** for 12 to 15 minutes, or until the centers are set. Let stand for 15 minutes to cool. Refrigerate for at least 2 hours. Just before serving, top each serving with a tablespoon of whipped topping. Dust with cocoa.

NUTRITIONAL INFO PER SERVING: 107 calories, 5 g protein, 21 g carbohydrates, 1 g fat (less than 1 g saturated), 2 g fiber, 149 mg sodium

CHOCOLATE-KAHLÚA MOUSSE PARFAITS

MAKES 4 SERVINGS

These parfaits are great when you want to entertain, yet still want to stick to your healthy way of life. Because of the sugar in the graham crackers and whipped topping, however, it's best not to make this an everyday treat. The layered combination of mousse, whipped topping, and graham cracker definitely makes this worth a splurge. Serve these desserts in wine glasses for a gorgeous presentation.

½ cup plus 1 tablespoon very cold fat-free milk

¼ cup Kahlúa or other coffee-flavored liqueur

1 envelope (1.5 ounces) sugar-free, low-fat chocolate mousse mix

1 tablespoon unsweetened cocoa powder

2 chocolate graham crackers, crushed into fine crumbs

1 cup thawed fat-free frozen whipped topping

1. **IN** a large mixing bowl, combine the milk, Kahlúa, mousse mix, and cocoa. With an electric mixer fitted with beaters, whip on low speed until blended. Slowly increase the mixer speed to high, whipping for 5 minutes, or until fluffy.

2. **IN** each of 4 large wine glasses or glass dessert bowls, layer ¼ cup of the mousse, 2 teaspoons of crumbs, and 2 tablespoons of topping. Repeat layering once more, using the remaining ingredients except for about ⅛ teaspoon of graham cracker crumbs. Sprinkle the top of each serving with a few of the remaining graham cracker crumbs.

3. **REFRIGERATE** for at least 2 hours before serving.

NUTRITIONAL INFO PER SERVING: 145 calories, 3 g protein, 22 g carbohydrates, 3 g fat (2 g saturated), 1 g fiber, 43 mg sodium

ICED BUFFED MOCHA

If you're guilty of hitting the nearest coffee empire for a chocolaty frozen coffee jolt, you're not alone. Not only will this recipe satisfy your craving in the privacy of your own home, it's likely to save you a significant amount of cash over time . . . oh, and fat and calories, too!

1 tablespoon water

¾ teaspoon instant coffee powder

1 cup light chocolate soy milk

2 tablespoons fat-free, artificially sweetened vanilla yogurt

1 packet (0.35 ounce) sugar substitute (such as Splenda)

8 ice cubes

2 tablespoons aerosol fat-free whipped topping (optional)

Cocoa powder (optional)

1. **IN** a small microwaveable cup, combine the water and coffee powder. Microwave on high power about 20 seconds, or until hot. Stir to dissolve the powder.

2. **IN** the jar of a blender, combine the milk, yogurt, sugar substitute, reserved coffee mixture, and ice. Blend on high speed or ice-crush setting for 30 to 60 seconds, or until smooth.

3. **POUR** into a large glass. Garnish with whipped topping and dust with cocoa, if desired. Serve immediately with a straw.

NUTRITIONAL INFO PER SERVING: 127 calories, 9 g protein, 18 g carbohydrates, 2 g fat (less than 1 g saturated), 1 g fiber, 223 mg sodium

HOW FAST WILL YOU LOSE?

You've heard that 2 pounds a week is safe, yet some contestants drop up to 10 times as much. What's healthy for you depends on your weight today.

Why can some contestants drop so much, so fast? The short answer is the more you weigh, the more you can safely lose when you start, says Michael Dansinger, MD, one of the show's medical experts. It boils down to simple math: Compare the number of calories you eat now with the number you should be eating to support your goal weight; the difference between the numbers is a calorie deficit—or the number of calories you need to cut per day to reach your goal. The more calories you need to cut, the more dramatic the results.

Find your current weight on the chart below to see how fast you'll lose, just by cutting calories.

IF YOU WEIGH (IN POUNDS)	YOU'RE CURRENTLY EATING ABOUT THIS MANY CALORIES JUST TO MAINTAIN YOUR WEIGHT	IF YOU CUT BACK TO 1,800 CALORIES PER DAY,* YOU CAN SAFELY LOSE ABOUT THIS MUCH A WEEK
400	5,200	7 pounds**
350	4,550	5.5
300	3,900	4.25
250	3,250	3
200	2,600	1.5
180	2,340	1
155	2,015	0.5
145	1,885	Less than 0.25

*An active woman can expect to reach a goal weight of about 135 pounds following a 1,800-calorie-a-day diet.
**Burn an extra 500 calories per day through exercise, and lose 1 more pound per week.

The Biggest Loser
EXERCISE PLAN

You can lose weight by dieting alone, but you can lose more weight faster—and get fit and healthier in the process—by adding exercise to the picture

The Biggest Loser diet formula is easy: Eat less, exercise more. It's really that simple. Now make it your mantra.

But let's be realistic. If dieting is hard, exercising can be even harder. For many folks, it's a matter of time, or lack thereof. Your day is already jam-packed: You rise and shine, maybe you get the kids off to school, you go to work, you come home, you make dinner, you help the kids with homework, you watch TV, and you go to bed. Exactly when are you supposed to fit in an hour of exercise? The answer is, you're just going to have to make it happen. No one else can do it for you—because not exercising is not an option.

Just like you have to give up certain foods to lose weight, you're going to have to give up certain things—some TV time or your lunch hour—to get fit. But trust us, the trade-off is worth it. After a while, it won't feel like a trade-off anymore,

Make sure that you check with your doctor before you start this or any exercise program.

because as soon as exercise becomes a part of your life, you won't be able to live without it. In fact, you won't be able to believe you ever lived without it.

HERE'S THE PLAN

Now you need to get started. But before you do, there are a few things to consider that might ease your fears. Remember, you are not a Biggest Loser cast member, so you don't have to exercise as rigorously as they do! We know that's not possible. The plan we provide here will work with your busy lifestyle. You'll be participating in both cardiovascular activity and circuit training, which includes weight lifting, strength training, and stretching.

If you sign on to the safe, healthy Biggest Loser diet and exercise plan, we promise that you will get in shape in less time than you thought possible. You need to devote at least 12 weeks to the plan for maximum results, but how long you stay on the plan will vary with your goals. And, clearly, we hope that a healthy diet and daily exercise will become part of your life forever.

Butt-Busting Cardio

The best way to burn calories and fat is with cardiovascular activity. That means you've got to shake your booty—you've got to move it to lose it! There are two ways to do just that, and you're going to do them both in the Biggest Loser cardio workout.

The Biggest Loser exercise plan starts with steady-state cardio. *Steady-state cardio* means that you'll get your heart rate in its fat-burning zone and keep it there for a specified amount of time at a set pace. Options include walking, jogging, running, swimming, biking, dancing, working out to a DVD, and using a cardio machine such as a treadmill, stair climber, stationary bicycle, or elliptical machine.

After you've gained a fitness base, you'll start to change it up with interval training. That means you'll alternate periods of high-intensity and low-intensity cardio activity. This method helps you burn more calories and fat, improves your cardiovascular fitness, and increases your speed.

Body-Sculpting Circuit Training

A circuit workout is a series of exercises (usually strength training) that you perform one right after another with only 5 to 8 seconds of rest in between. In circuit training, you'll alternate muscle groups, starting with one, then progressing to another. This approach creates body-firming muscle and increases aerobic capacity, all while reducing body fat. Because you'll perform in time intervals, you'll need a clock or a watch with a second hand to time yourself. You can also wear a heart rate monitor to monitor your heart rate in the fat-burning zone.

The Biggest Loser circuit training workout will look familiar to you, as it includes push-ups, squats, shoulder presses, bicep curls, lunges, chair dips, dumbbell rows, and abdominal crunches. Begin all circuit routines with 5 minutes of walking, marching, or jogging in place, and be sure to stretch and cool down.

We recommend performing circuit training three times each week, resting at least a day between workouts.

Do More, Lose More, Look Better

If you have extra time, consider complementing your cardio and circuit workouts with other forms of exercise. If you play tennis, racquetball, volleyball, basketball, or if you like to dance, you'll complement your conventional cardio by engaging in intense bursts of muscle activity. Yoga and Pilates also will complement your circuit by concentrating on building inner strength, core strength, and flexibility, and by teaching you proper breathing. Remember, the more you do, the more you lose! By burning 250 to 500 calories a day through exercise, you could lose up to a whole pound a week. So get to it!

Part 3

FITNESS
MOVES

CHAPTER 10

The Years-Off WORKOUT

Breakthrough science! Get up to 10 pounds lighter and take 10 years off your body with our three-part age-defying plan

You already know exercise makes you look and feel younger. But here's a news flash: Exercise actually does make you younger—right down to your DNA. When researchers examined the lifestyle habits and DNA of more than 2,400 twins, they found that regular exercisers had significantly longer telomeres (a region of DNA that acts as a biological marker for aging) than their sedentary peers. Those who exercised a little less than 30 minutes a day had telomeres that looked 10 years younger than those who did just 16 minutes a week.

Ready to roll back the years? Our age-defying plan includes all the elements you need to get slimmer and feel younger—total-body strength, high-energy cardio, and stress-busting yoga. Combine this with our "Foods That Fight Fat" in Chapter 7. Try our plan for 8 weeks, and you'll drop up to two dress or waist sizes while boosting your health.

PROGRAM AT A GLANCE

Here's what a week's worth of workouts would look like. You can do the cardio, sculpt, or yoga sessions back-to-back or split them up. For example, do 10 minutes of yoga in the AM, then your cardio and/or sculpt in the PM.

★ MONDAY: Cardio Intervals 40 minutes, Yoga 10 minutes

★ TUESDAY: Sculpt 20 minutes, Cardio 25 to 50 minutes, Yoga 10 minutes

★ WEDNESDAY: Yoga 10 minutes

★ THURSDAY: Sculpt 20 minutes, Cardio 25 to 50 minutes, Yoga 10 minutes

★ FRIDAY: Cardio Intervals 40 minutes, Yoga 10 minutes

★ SATURDAY: Sculpt 20 minutes, Cardio 25 to 50 minutes, Yoga 10 minutes

★ SUNDAY: Cardio 25 to 50 minutes, Yoga 10 minutes

This plan was designed by Mubarakah Ibrahim, owner of Balance Fitness in New Haven, Connecticut, a women-only personal training facility.

PART 1: YEARS-OFF SCULPTING

Why it works: Starting at about age 40, your metabolism slows by roughly 5 percent each decade. By age 50, you'll have gained about 10 pounds of fat and lost 5 pounds of muscle.

Lifting weights counters this decline, boosting metabolism by about 7 percent, which burns about 100 extra calories a day. And the workout itself has an afterburn effect, which burns even more fat.

A recent study found that women who strength-trained kept their metabolism revved about 2 hours postworkout, for a bonus burn of about 130 calories. Plus, exercise promotes the conversion of testosterone to estrogen in muscles, so you maintain higher estrogen levels, which helps keep midlife belly fat at bay.

With more muscle, you'll also have more energy. "Often women will say, 'I used to garden,' or 'I used to dance,' but they've lost their strength," says Ibrahim. "Strength-training turns the tide."

Do 3 sets of 10 reps. Pick the level that suits you best: If the main move feels too hard, try the easier variation. If it's too easy, add more weight.

How often: 3 days a week (20 minutes)

What you'll need: A workout mat, a low step (or staircase step or table), and 5- to 10-pound dumbbells. If that weight feels easy to lift by the end of each set, use a heavier one.

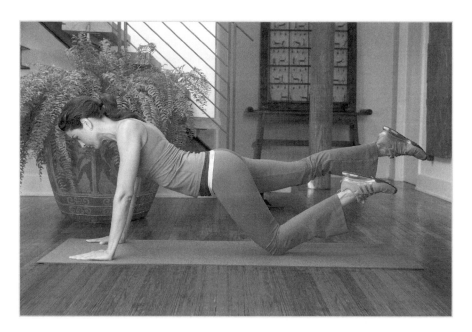

⌃ PUSH-UP KICK-BACK

FIRMS CHEST, SHOULDERS, BACK, GLUTES

Begin in a modified push-up position with hands on floor slightly more than shoulder-width apart and knees bent, forming a straight line from shoulders to knees. Bend arms and lower chest until upper arms are parallel to floor. Press back up and extend right leg straight back, toes pointed, squeezing glutes (pictured). Return to start. Repeat push-up, this time extending left leg. Continue, alternating legs. To make it harder, just do a full push-up.

MAKE IT EASIER: Eliminate the leg extension.

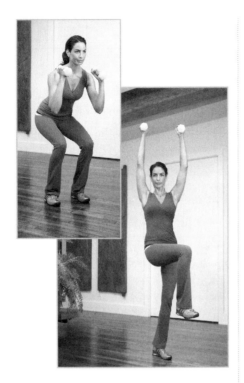

⊘ SQUAT TWIST AND LIFT

FIRMS SHOULDERS, ARMS, ABDOMINALS, OBLIQUES, GLUTES, THIGHS

Stand with feet shoulder-width apart. Hold weights at shoulder height, elbows down and palms facing in. Bend knees and squat as if sitting into a chair, keeping knees behind toes, until thighs are nearly parallel to floor. Stand up, pressing weights overhead while turning torso about 45 degrees to the right, lifting right knee forward to hip height. Return to start; switch sides and repeat, lifting left knee and turning torso to left. Continue, alternating sides with each rep.

MAKE IT EASIER: Keep weights at shoulders; lift knee only halfway.

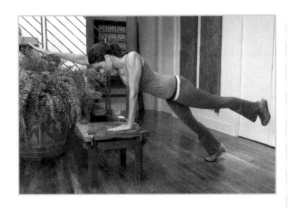

⊘ SUPERWOMAN IN FLIGHT

FIRMS BACK, CORE

Begin in a full push-up position, hands on a table or low step directly beneath shoulders, feet on floor about hip-width apart. Raise right arm forward to shoulder height while lifting left foot behind you. Return to start and repeat, this time reaching left arm forward and right leg back.

MAKE IT EASIER: Do the move with hands on a countertop-high surface.

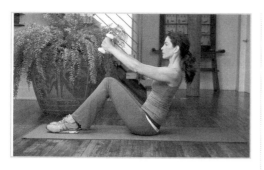

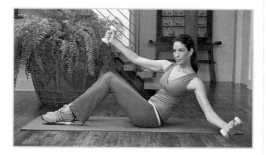

⟨ SINGLE-ARM V-FLY

FIRMS ABS, OBLIQUES

Sit on floor with back straight, leaning back slightly, knees bent, and feet flat on floor. Hold a dumbbell in each hand with elbows slightly bent, arms forward with palms facing each other. Keeping back straight, lower torso about halfway to floor. Rotate torso to the left, lowering left hand out to side and toward floor with elbow slightly bent; keep right arm at center. Return to start; repeat move to opposite side.

MAKE IT EASIER: Bring weights straight out to sides; don't twist torso.

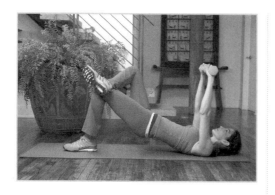

⟨ CHEST AND BUTT PRESS

FIRMS CHEST, ARMS, SHOULDERS, GLUTES

Lie faceup on floor, knees bent, right ankle crossed over left knee. Hold weights at chest level, elbows bent 90 degrees, palms facing forward. Squeeze glutes and lift hips a few inches off the floor while pressing weights toward ceiling. Return to start. Perform half a set, then switch legs.

MAKE IT EASIER: Keep both feet on floor.

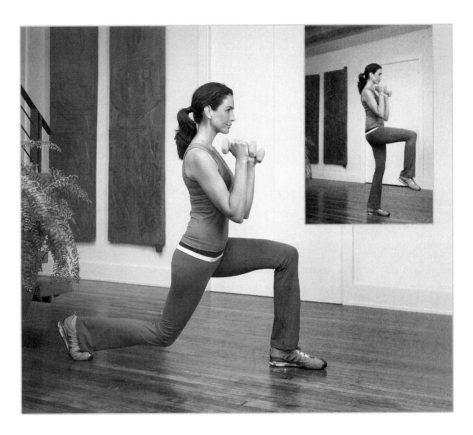

⌃HAMMER-CURL LUNGE

FIRMS GLUTES, THIGHS, BICEPS

Stand with feet hip-width apart. Hold a dumbbell in each hand with arms at sides, palms facing in. Take a giant step back with right leg, bending both knees until left thigh is parallel to floor, keeping left knee behind toes. At the same time, curl weights to shoulders, keeping elbows close to body. Stand back up, lifting right knee forward to hip height. Lower arms and return to starting position; switch sides.

MAKE IT EASIER: Hold lunge position and just do curls (no knee lift); switch legs halfway through set.

See it live! Follow along with Chris Freytag as she demonstrates all the fat-burning and muscle-firming moves at prevention.com/blastfat.

PART 2: INCHES-OFF CARDIO

Why it works: As you enter into your 40s and beyond, your estrogen levels dip, leaving you with more testosterone and the traditionally male-patterned weight gain around the middle that comes with it. To fight this common middle-age spread, you need to make at least two of your weekly cardio workouts an interval routine, combining bursts of intensity and recovery.

This is supported by good science: Canadian researchers found that just 2 weeks of alternate-day interval training boosted active women's fat-burning ability by 36 percent.

"When you push your body, it responds by quickly increasing your ability to deliver blood to working muscles and to use oxygen and burn fat, in case you make it work that hard again," explains Martin Gibala, PhD, associate professor of kinesiology at McMaster University. Plus, intervals might help counter age-related health concerns: Researchers from Norway found that doing intervals reduced blood pressure, controlled blood sugar, and improved HDL (good) cholesterol.

What to Do

Six days a week, pick an aerobic workout from our high-energy activities list (page 180) to burn about 450 calories. Make two of these workouts an interval routine (see "Intervals Made Easy," below). For the remaining 4 days, do some form of steady-paced aerobic exercise for 25 to 50 minutes to burn fat and stay fit.

How often: 6 days a week (25 to 50 minutes)

Intervals Made Easy

Boost your calorie burn while turning back the clock with intervals. We've given a suggested treadmill routine, but you can do it with any cardio workout—just increase the intensity for the prescribed amount of time. Use your rate of perceived exertion (RPE; how difficult the activity feels on a scale of 1 to 10) to determine your pace.

TIME	EFFORT	PACE	RPE
0–3 minutes	Warm up, working up to brisk pace	3.0–3.5 mph	3–4
4–10 minutes	Brisk walk	3.5–4.0 mph	5–6
11–12 minutes	Walk very briskly or jog	4.1–6.0 mph	7–8
13–15 minutes	Brisk walk	3.5–4.0 mph	5–6
16–35 minutes	Repeat minutes 11–15 four more times, walking very briskly or jogging for 2 minutes and recovering at a moderately brisk pace for 3 minutes		
36–40 minutes	Cool down, slowing to an easy pace	3.0–3.5 mph	3–4

BURN 450 CALORIES!

Pick Your Activity

EXERCISE	TIME (MINUTES)
Aerobics class	40
Cycling outdoors (moderate, at 12 mph)	35
Cycling (stationary)	40
Dance Yourself Thin (*Prevention* DVD)	40
Elliptical machine	30
Inline skating	25
Jogging	30
Step machine	30
Swimming laps freestyle	40
Tennis	40
Walking (4.0 mph)	50
Walk-jogging	45 (includes 5–10 minutes total jogging time)

Calorie counts are based on a 150-pound person. Each workout burns about 300 calories, plus an extra 150-calorie "afterburn"—the calories you continue to burn postexercise, according to researchers.

PART 3: STRESS-OFF YOGA

Why it works: Stress is one of the biggest contributors to the aging process, robbing you of precious sleep, increasing harmful inflammation, damaging your DNA, and even causing wrinkles.

But yoga can be one of your best stress-busters: Recent studies have shown that yoga reduces markers of oxidative stress, a condition that can accelerate damage linked to aging. Yoga also improves flexibility, which deteriorates over time as the tissues that support your joints stiffen, and relieves back pain, so you move more easily.

Here's the best news: You don't need a ton of time to reap these rewards, so long as you stay consistent. Daily yoga practice—even just 10 minutes—carries a greater benefit than a weekly class because you're fighting that stress a little at a time, says Carol Krucoff, a yoga therapist with Duke Integrative Medicine in Durham, North Carolina, and creator of the CD *Healing Moves Yoga*.

Do it first thing in the morning, she adds, and you'll increase energy, release tension, and start the day off right.

What to Do

The moves in the following 10-minute routine are scientifically shown to fight stress. For each pose, inhale slowly and deeply through your nose for 5 seconds, and then exhale slowly for another 5. Try to clear your mind and allow yourself to focus on nothing but your breath moving through your body. Repeat this breathing pattern 3 to 6 times, and then move to the next pose.

How often: Daily (It's only 10 minutes!)

What you'll need: A workout mat, yoga block or phone book, and if you'd like, grab some folded bath towels or blankets for your comfort.

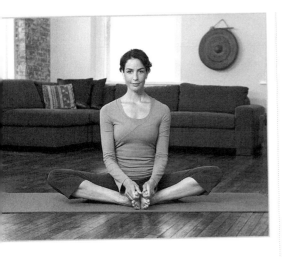

⊙ BOUND ANGLE POSE

STRETCHES INNER THIGHS AND GROIN MUSCLES; TRADITIONALLY THOUGHT TO SOOTHE MENOPAUSE SYMPTOMS; REDUCES FATIGUE

Sit tall with soles of feet together, knees bent out to sides. Bring heels as close to pelvis as comfortably possible. Grasp big toe of each foot with first and second fingers and thumb; hold here, sitting tall.

MAKE IT EASIER: Place some thickly folded towels or blankets under each thigh for additional support.

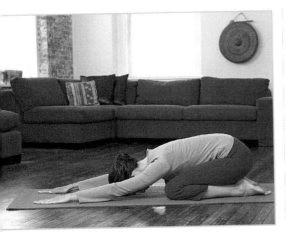

⊙ CHILD'S POSE

STRETCHES HIPS, THIGHS, BACK

From a kneeling position, sit back on heels and open knees about hip-width. Bend forward, lowering upper body between thighs and forehead toward floor; bring arms in front of body, palms down.

MAKE IT EASIER: Place a thickly folded towel or blanket between your calves and hamstrings.

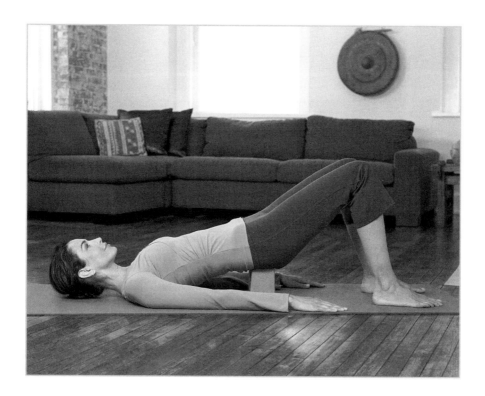

⌃ SUPPORTED BRIDGE

STRETCHES SPINE, CHEST, ABDOMEN; RELAXES LOWER BACK

Lie on back with knees bent, feet flat on floor, and arms at sides with palms down. Press into soles of feet and lift hips. Slide yoga block under tailbone, and then allow body to rest on block. Remain here, breathing evenly. To come out of the pose, press into feet, lift hips, remove block, lower back to floor, and then gently roll up to a seated position.

MAKE IT EASIER: Use a lower part of the block or substitute a phone book for the yoga block.

CHAPTER 11

SHRINK YOUR BELLY IN 14 DAYS!

The research is in! Our fastest-ever routine will firm and flatten you from all angles in just 2 weeks

We have some really great news for your abs: The über-ultimate piece of belly flab-busting equipment is a $30 stability ball. When researchers at California State University, Sacramento, hooked up electrodes to the midsections of 18 people, they found that ball moves recruited twice the number of muscle fibers as traditional crunches or yoga/Pilates-inspired workouts.

Scientists credit the ball's instability with doubling the toning power of these moves. To amp up results, we combined ball exercises from the study with high-energy cardio and simple calorie-cutting tips. In 2 weeks, you could lose up to an inch from your waist; in 4 weeks, shed up to 8 pounds or even more.

These workouts were designed by Rafael Escamilla, PhD, PT, study author and professor of physical therapy at California State University, Sacramento, and Wayne L. Westcott, PhD, exercise science coordinator at Quincy College in Massachusetts.

PROGRAM AT A GLANCE
Here's your workout plan.

Week 1

★ MONDAY: Cardio (page 193) Routine 1 (45 to 60 minutes)

★ TUESDAY: Belly Workout (opposite page) (once, 25 to 30 minutes)

★ WEDNESDAY: Cardio Routine 2 (35 to 45 minutes)

★ THURSDAY: Belly Workout (once, 25 to 30 minutes)

★ FRIDAY: Cardio Routine 1 (45 to 60 minutes)

★ SATURDAY: Belly Workout (once, 25 to 30 minutes)

★ SUNDAY: Cardio Routine 2 (35 to 45 minutes)

Week 2

★ MONDAY: Belly Workout (twice, 45 to 50 minutes)

★ TUESDAY: Cardio Routine 1 (45 to 60 minutes)

★ WEDNESDAY: Belly Workout (twice, 45 to 50 minutes)

★ THURSDAY: Cardio Routine 2 (35 to 45 minutes)

★ FRIDAY: Belly Workout (45 to 50 minutes)

★ SATURDAY: Cardio Routine 1 (45 to 60 minutes)

★ SUNDAY: Belly Workout (twice, 45 to 50 minutes)

Combine this workout with "Foods That Fight Fat" in Chapter 7 for the fastest results. The simple food swaps cut about 500 calories from your diet daily. Our recommendations also boost your intake of monounsaturated fatty acids (MUFAs) and whole grains. Studies show both shrink belly fat faster.

Do 12 to 15 reps of each move. Between each exercise, do a cardio burst—2 minutes of jumping rope, marching or jogging in place, stair climbing or stepping, or doing jumping jacks. Remember to warm up and cool down by marching or stepping side to side in place for 3 to 5 minutes at the beginning and end of your workout. These 2-minute high-energy cardio bursts will double your calorie burn to speed up fat loss and reveal a slimmer belly in less time.

BELLY WORKOUT

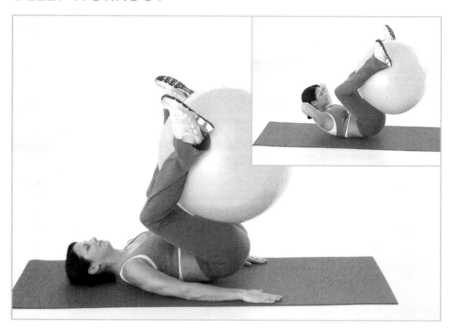

⌃ REVERSE CRUNCH

Lie faceup with calves resting on ball, arms at sides. Press legs into ball, squeezing it between calves and thighs. Contract abs and lift hips 3 to 6 inches off floor and pull knees toward chest. Hold for 1 second, then lower. Then do a cardio burst for 2 minutes.

MAKE IT EASIER: Contract abs and just lift ball off floor, keeping hips down.

MAKE IT HARDER: Keeping neck in line with spine, l;ead and shoulders off floor as you raise hips. Hold, then lower both upper body and hips.

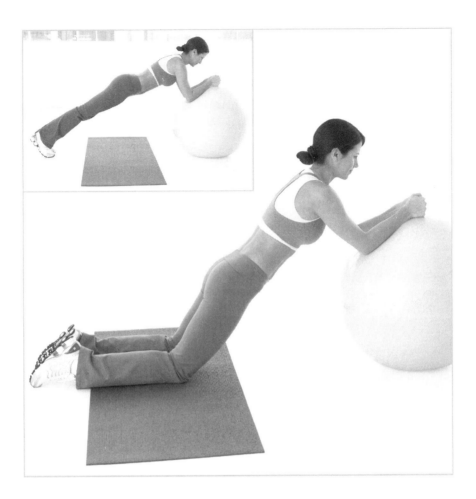

⌃ ROCK AND ROLL

Start on knees, with legs about hip-width apart. Place fists on ball in front of you. Keeping body in line from head to knees and abs tight, lean forward and roll onto forearms. Hold for 1 second, then roll back to start. Then do a cardio burst for 2 minutes.

MAKE IT EASIER: Bend hips instead of keeping body in a straight line as you roll onto forearms, or keep body in line and roll only partway onto forearms.

MAKE IT HARDER: Once you're balancing on forearms, straighten legs and press balls of feet into floor to form a straight line from head to heels. Hold for 15 to 30 seconds and repeat.

LAB-TESTED BELLY FLATTENERS

For a firm, flat belly, think outside the crunch: Experts say the best moves are those that engage the deepest stomach muscles to pull in your waistline like a corset. Researcher Michele Olson, PhD, an exercise physiologist at Auburn University, found that the following two moves were tops in targeting the key muscles. Do them 3 times a week.

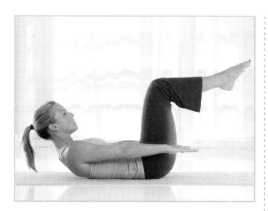

ⓧ THE HUNDRED

Lie on back with arms at sides, palms down, knees bent to 90 degrees. Raise head, lifting upper back and arms a few inches, and engage abs. Inhale as you pulse arms up and down an inch to a count of 5; exhale for 5 pulses. Do 10 times, for a total of 100 pulses.

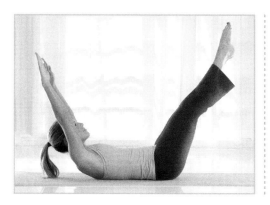

ⓧ DOUBLE LEG STRETCH

Still on back, lift shoulder blades, engage abs, exhale, and hug knees toward chest, hands on shins. Inhale and extend legs forward while bringing arms back, forming a big V. Return knees to chest; repeat 8 to 10 times.

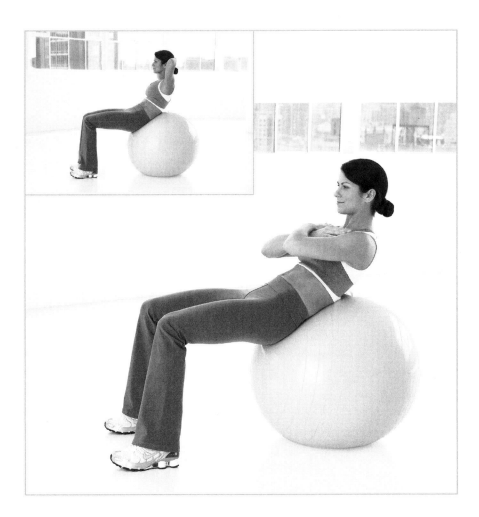

⋀ BALL CURL

Sit on ball, walk feet forward, and roll torso down until bottom of butt is just off ball and middle and lower back are on ball, feet together. Place hands behind head. Lean back, pressing upper back into ball, then exhale, contract abs, and curl forward until upper back lifts off ball. Then do a cardio burst for 2 minutes.

MAKE IT EASIER: Place feet wider than hip-width apart for more stability, and cross arms over chest.

MAKE IT HARDER: Straighten one leg so it's parallel to floor and you're balancing on one foot. Do half the repetitions, then switch legs to finish.

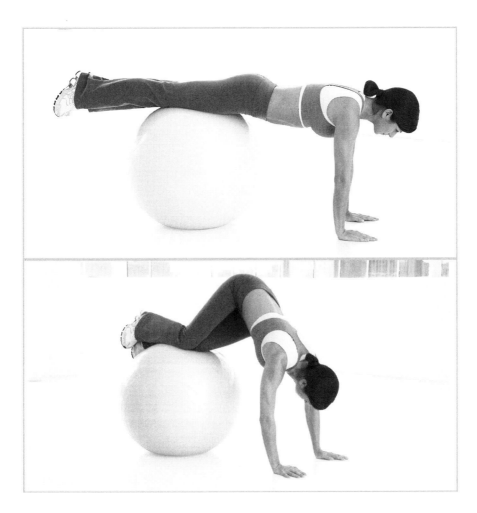

⌃ SKIER

Lie over ball on all fours. Walk hands forward so ball rolls under thighs, legs together, abs tight, and body in line from head to toes. Bend knees and pull them and ball (it will roll to shins) toward right shoulder. Hold for 1 second, then roll back out and repeat to left side. Then do a cardio burst for 2 minutes.

MAKE IT EASIER: Hold start position—body in line from head to toes, abs contracted—for 15 to 30 seconds. Repeat one more time.

MAKE IT HARDER: Start with ball under shins and let it roll to tops of feet as you draw knees in.

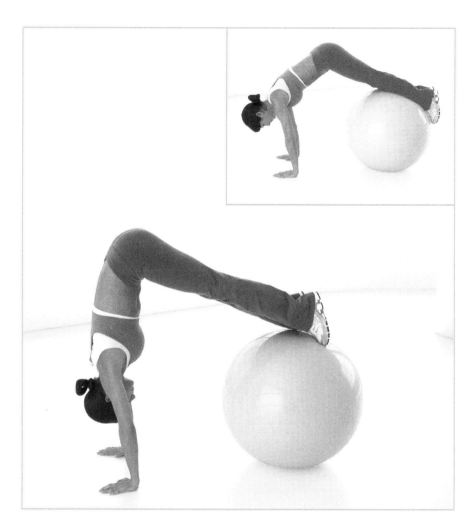

⌃ PIKE

Start in the same position as the Skier, legs together, ball under thighs, balancing on hands, and body in line from head to toes. Keeping legs straight, contract abs and lift hips up toward ceiling, rolling ball to shins. Hold for 1 second, then lower. Then do a cardio burst for 2 minutes.

MAKE IT EASIER: Lift hips just a few inches and roll ball to about knees.

MAKE IT HARDER: Start with ball under shins and roll to tops of feet and lift hips so torso is as vertical as possible, like you're doing a handstand.

CARDIO ROUTINES

The following calorie-melting workouts maximize fat loss, boost your energy, and improve your fitness level—fast! In one study, dieters who also walked 50 minutes 3 times a week lost nearly twice as much belly fat as women who only dieted. You can do any type of cardio exercise (walking, jogging, cycling, or using a cardio machine) with these workouts.

Routine 1

★ Burns 225 to 675 calories, for a 150-pound person.

★ Warm up at an easy pace for 3 minutes, then exercise at a moderate to brisk pace (breathing hard but still able to talk in sentences) for 40 to 55 minutes, and cool down at an easy pace for 2 minutes.

★ **Total time:** 45 to 60 minutes

Routine 2

★ Burns 175 to 500 calories, for a 150-pound person.

★ Warm up for 3 minutes, then pick it up to a moderate to brisk intensity for 3 minutes, then push yourself to go as fast as you can for 2 minutes (able to speak only a few words at a time). Alternate brisk and fast intervals 5 to 7 more times, then cool down for 2 minutes.

★ **Total time:** 35 to 45 minutes

HOW TO BUY A BALL

Most people need a 22-inch (or 55-cm) stability ball. If you're under 5-foot-1, choose an 18-inch (or 45-cm) one, or a 26-inch (or 65-cm) ball if 5-foot-8 or taller. They're available in sporting goods stores (about $30) or online.

We like the Gymnic Plus (performbetter.com) because it's made with burst-resistant, latex-free vinyl, and if punctured, it will deflate slowly.

PREVENTION Alert!

BARGAIN AB FLATTENER

Surprise: The #1 gadget for a sexy belly isn't sold on late-night TV!

Yes, we love stability balls. But a new study shows they're not the *only* way to firm your belly. When Northern Illinois University researchers sized up ab moves done on an inflatable disk, stability ball, Bosu trainer, and bench, the disks took first prize, activating an average of 24 percent more muscle fiber than the others. Researchers say balancing on the disk's 13-inch surface had a tightropelike effect.

Better yet, at under $25, the disk was also the cheapest solution tested. (VersaDisc; power-systems.com)

BEST BELLY ALL-AROUND

Slim down your middle faster with this dual routine that tones both your belly and back in one shot. Although some ab exercises can strain your spine—even if you don't feel pain when you do them—these isometric moves, in which you hold a position instead of doing lots of reps, were proven in an exercise lab to firm the midsection with minimal stress to the lower back. Plus, a stronger back improves your posture, giving you an instant tummy tuck. Get started now to see results in 3 weeks.

This workout was designed by Stuart McGill, PhD, author of *Ultimate Back Fitness and Performance* and a professor of spine biomechanics at the University of Waterloo in Canada.

What to do: Perform the moves in the order listed. Hold each for 10 seconds, bracing your abs (as though a ball were going to hit you in the stomach), but don't hold your breath. Repeat 4 to 8 times. Try the main move first. If it's too difficult, do the Make It Easier option. When you can complete 8 reps of the main move with ease, progress to the Make It Harder version. Do this 15-minute routine once a day, at least an hour after you wake up, so your muscles are warm.

For faster results: Do 30 minutes of cardio, such as walking, jogging, or cycling, most days, with 1 long, 60- to 90-minute workout each week.

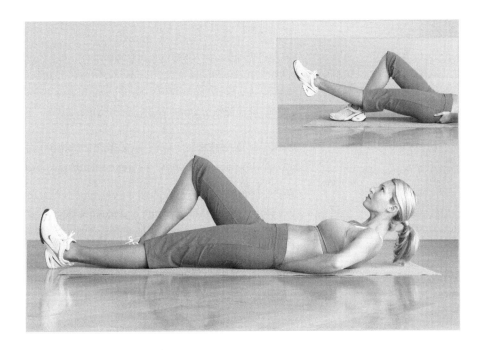

⌃ CONTROLLED STATIC CURL

Lie with right knee bent, foot flat on floor, left leg extended, hands under lower back. Lift elbows and inhale deeply. As you exhale, contract abs and curl head, neck, and shoulders to raise shoulder blades a few inches off floor. Hold and lower, including elbows. Do all reps, then switch legs.

MAKE IT EASIER: Simply brace abs, hold, then release, keeping head on floor.

MAKE IT HARDER: Lift extended leg a few inches off floor and hold as you raise and lower upper body. Switch legs and repeat.

FLAT BELLY AFTER 40!

You'll get quicker results if you're using good technique. For video demos of the exercises and advice on proper form, go to prevention.com/ballworkout.

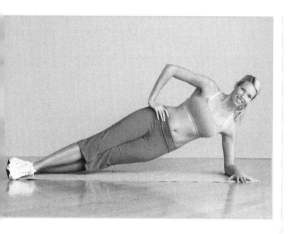

⊙ SIDE BRIDGE

Lie on left side, propped up on elbow, with top foot in front of bottom so both feet are on floor. Contract abs as you raise body, forming a straight line from toes to shoulders. Do all reps, then switch sides.

MAKE IT EASIER: Lie with legs bent behind you and raise torso and thighs, resting on bottom knee.

MAKE IT HARDER: From main move, rotate body to face floor, supporting yourself on forearms and toes, legs and torso in a straight line. Hold, then rotate back to Side Bridge. Do all reps, then switch sides.

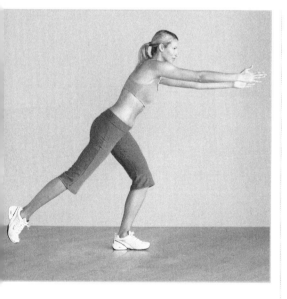

⊙ ONE-LEGGED SQUAT

Stand with right leg extended behind you, toes on floor. Hold arms out to sides at shoulder height. With abs contracted, bend left knee about 45 degrees, hinging forward a bit from hips, and slide right leg back as arms press forward, palms facing in. (Keep left knee behind toes.) Lift right leg slightly (1 to 2 inches, as pictured) and hold. Straighten left leg to stand, returning right leg to start and pressing arms back out to sides. Do all reps, then switch legs.

MAKE IT EASIER: Keep back toe on floor throughout move.

MAKE IT HARDER: Raise right leg higher (3 to 6 inches) when you extend it behind you, and keep it lifted throughout the entire move.

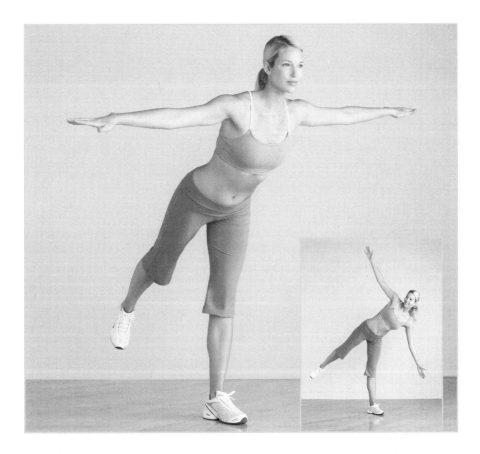

⌃ HIP AIRPLANE

Stand with right leg extended behind you so foot is off floor. Raise arms to shoulder height like wings, palms down. Contract abs and hinge torso forward about 45 degrees as you raise right leg behind you as high as possible, while maintaining balance and keeping hips level. Hold, then lower leg to stand and repeat. Do all reps, then switch legs.

MAKE IT EASIER: Lift your leg behind your body and balance without hinging forward with your upper body.

MAKE IT HARDER: From main move, rotate body to right, raising right arm so chest and hips face right and left arm points toward floor (shown). Hold, then rotate to left. Hold and return to center for 1 repetition. Do all reps, then repeat with opposite leg lifted.

CHAPTER 12

TONE YOUR ARMS— IN 10 MINUTES!

Bare your arms with confidence in
4 weeks with this targeted routine

Shapely, sculpted arms are possible—at any age. All it takes is this 10-minute routine, which you can tailor to your fitness level. These four firming moves work the chest, shoulders, and arms from every angle to tighten and tone the droopiness that can start when you lose lean tissue in your 40s. After a month, you'll be on your way to show-off arms that will look great all year long.

WORKOUT AT A GLANCE

What you need: 3- to 5-pound and 8- to 10-pound dumbbells and a mat or carpeted space

How to do it: Perform the routine 2 or 3 times a week on nonconsecutive days. Begin with a 5-minute dynamic warm-up: March in place while scissoring arms overhead (such as jumping jacks). For each exercise, do 2 sets of 10 to 12 reps (or 10 on each side, if appropriate). Rest 30 seconds in between sets.

Begin with the main move. If it's too difficult, do the Make It Easier option. Not challenging enough? Try the Make It Harder variation.

For quicker results: Do 3 sets and add 30 minutes of cardio, such as walking, cycling, or swimming, 3 to 5 days a week.

The expert: Kate Moran, a master trainer at Equinox fitness center in Chicago, has helped dozens of women sculpt their upper bodies.

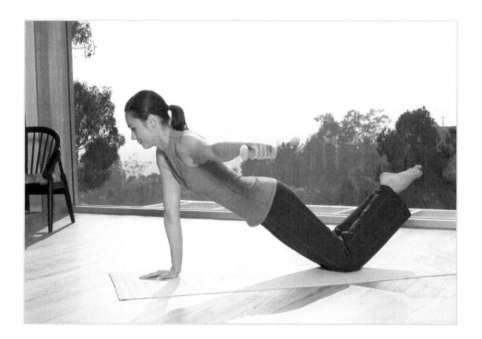

⊙ STARFISH

Get into push-up position on knees, hands directly beneath shoulders with light dumbbell in left hand. Engaging abs to stabilize torso, raise left arm straight out to side, parallel to floor. Hold for a second, then slowly lower to start and repeat. Do all reps, then switch arms.

MAKE IT EASIER: Ditch the dumbbell.

MAKE IT HARDER: Bring your knees off mat so you're balancing on toes and hands as you do the reps.

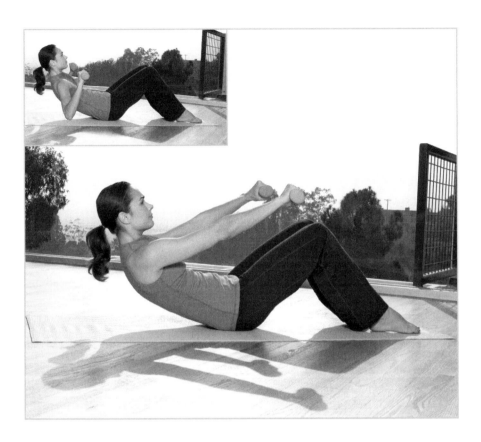

⌃ SIT-UP PULLOVER

Lie faceup on floor, knees bent, feet flat, and arms extended overhead with a light dumbbell in each hand. Contract abs and slowly curl up, lifting head, shoulders, and back off floor. Simultaneously bring arms forward in an arc toward knees. Hold for a second, then slowly reverse to start.

MAKE IT EASIER: Keep head on floor as you raise dumbbells in an arc and bring them down to floor so arms rest at sides. Reverse to start.

MAKE IT HARDER: Add a chest press. With upper body lifted and arms in front of you, bend elbows and lower dumbbells toward chest, then straighten arms before returning to start.

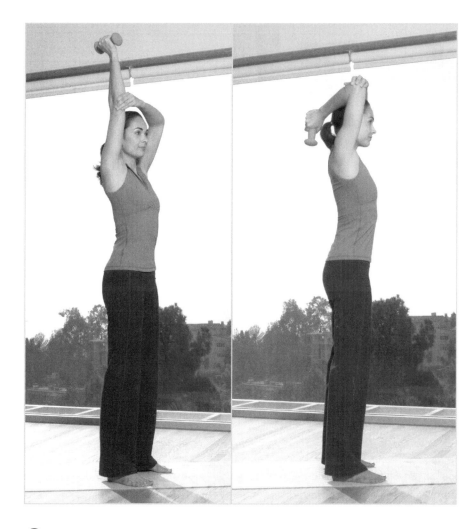

⌃ PONYTAIL EXTENSIONS

Stand with feet hip-width apart. Hold light dumbbell in right hand, arm extended straight overhead, left hand supporting right elbow to prevent it from flaring out. Bend elbow, lowering dumbbell behind head, then press back up to start position. Do all reps, then repeat on opposite side.

MAKE IT EASIER: Hold the ends of a single dumbbell with each hand so it's horizontal to work both arms at the same time.

MAKE IT HARDER: Use the heavier dumbbell.

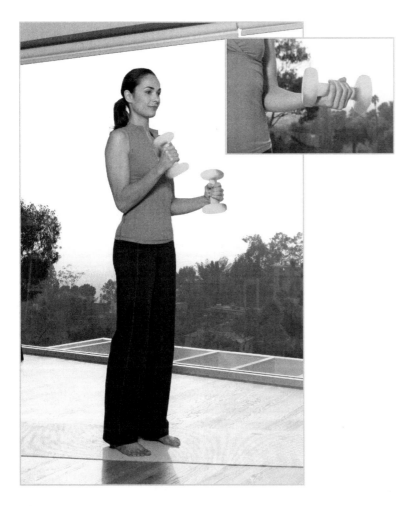

⌃ HANDBAG CURL

Stand with feet shoulder-width apart, arms at sides, a heavy dumbbell in each hand, palms facing in. Bend left arm to 90 degrees, dumbbell vertical. Hold that position as you bend right arm and curl dumbbell to shoulder, keeping elbow in to side. Complete all reps, then lower both arms and repeat, holding right arm at 90 degrees.

MAKE IT EASIER: Alternate curling each arm up to shoulder without holding either arm stationary.

MAKE IT HARDER: Hold dumbbell in the stationary hand with palm facing up so it's horizontal rather than vertical.

CHAPTER 13

Award-Winning BUTT MOVES

Here are the four absolute best toning exercises, based on new research

Frustrated by your butt? We discovered brand-new research from the University of North Carolina that revealed the most effective moves for sculpting a sexy, shapely backside. In fact, the exercises in this 10-minute routine beat out the competition by activating muscles up to 30 percent more than traditional moves.

Add in regular cardio 4 to 5 times a week, and researchers say you'll start noticing a firmer, shapelier rear in as little as 2 to 4 weeks. Bonus: Since a strong backside powers just about everything you do, from hiking up stairs to rushing through errands, you'll feel more energized all day long.

This workout was designed by Lindsay DiStefano, a certified athletic trainer, who is completing a doctorate in human movement science at the University of North Carolina.

WORKOUT AT A GLANCE

What you need: A medium resistance band ($5; spriproducts.com); optional: a set of 5- to 10-pound dumbbells and a chair

How to do it: Do 8 to 12 repetitions of each exercise on each side. Do the entire routine twice through 3 times a week on nonconsecutive days.

Try the main move first. If it's too difficult, do the Make It Easier option. For more of a challenge, try the Make It Harder version.

For quicker results: Do 3 sets of 10 to 15 reps every other day, and also add in 30 to 60 minutes of cardio, such as walking, jogging, or cycling, on most days of the week.

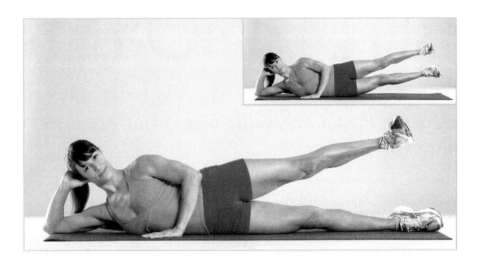

⌃ SIDE LEG LIFTS

Lie on right side with legs stacked, right arm bent and head supported on right hand, left hand resting on floor in front of chest for balance. Raise left leg about 2 feet, keeping foot flexed and squeezing butt. Pause, then slowly lower. Complete all reps, then switch sides.

MAKE IT EASIER: Bend top leg to 90 degrees, and lift with leg bent.

MAKE IT HARDER: Double up: Once top leg is lifted, raise bottom leg to meet top leg, pause, and then lower one leg at a time.

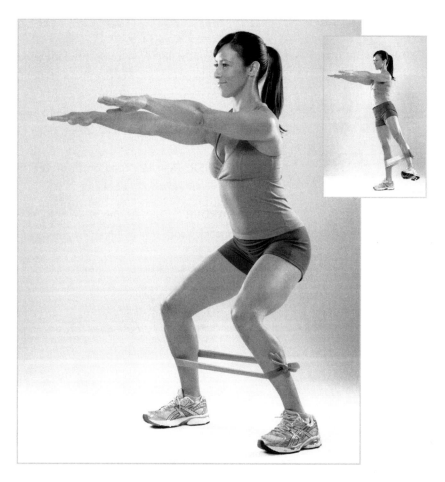

⌃ BANDED SHUFFLE

Stand with feet a few inches apart, and tie elastic band in taut loop around shins, hands extended to front at shoulder level. Step about 3 feet to right, then bend knees and sit back until thighs are almost parallel to floor, keeping knees behind toes. Staying low, step left foot to follow. Take two more shuffle steps to right, then switch directions and repeat.

MAKE IT EASIER: After stepping with right foot, stand and lift left leg to side for a balance challenge. Repeat toward left, lifting right foot for a side lift.

MAKE IT HARDER: Bend knees only 45 degrees, and step out just slightly more than hip-width.

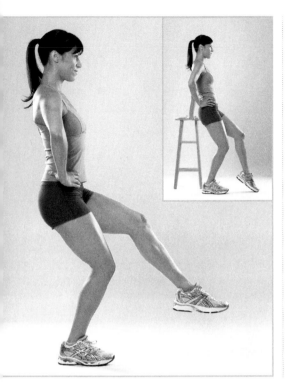

< BALANCING SQUAT

Balance on right foot, left knee bent with foot lifted a few inches off floor in front. Keeping back straight, slowly sit back into right leg, bending right knee about 45 degrees. Pause, then press into right heel to stand up. Complete all reps, then switch sides.

MAKE IT EASIER: Rest left toes on floor and, if needed, use a chair or stool for balance.

MAKE IT HARDER: Complete the move holding a dumbbell in each hand.

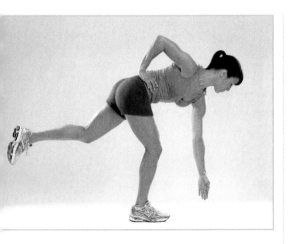

< SINGLE LEG DEADLIFT

Balance on right foot, with knee soft and hands on hips, left leg lifted behind. With abs tight and back straight, hinge forward from hips, lowering left hand toward right foot. Pull through right leg to return to standing. Do all reps on right leg; switch sides.

MAKE IT EASIER: Rest hand on back of chair for balance.

MAKE IT HARDER: Reach both hands to floor, dumbbell in each hand.

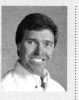

SOUND ADVICE

THE TOP THREE EXERCISES TO DO WHILE BRUSHING YOUR TEETH

We asked Wayne L. Westcott, PhD, exercise science coordinator at Quincy College in Massachusetts, for three simple exercises to do while brushing your teeth—multitasking at its best. Here's what he suggests.

1. CALF RAISES: Work out your calf muscles and your gluteal muscle by rising up on your toes and contracting your butt muscles, and then lowering back down to the floor, says Dr. Westcott. Do this 8 to 12 times. It takes about 60 seconds.

2. LEG STRETCH: Take a wide stance, with your feet more than shoulder-width apart. Then bend your left knee and stretch toward your left, feeling the stretch in the inner thigh of your right leg. Hold the stretch for at least 10 seconds. Stand back up and then bend your right knee and stretch to your right, stretching the inner thigh area of your left leg. This is a very good stretch, and most people don't stretch those areas, Dr. Westcott says. You can repeat the stretch two or three times.

3. SIDE STRETCH: If you brush your teeth with your right hand, put your left arm over your head and stretch to your right. Hold the stretch for at least 10 seconds. This stretches the muscles in your rib cage and under your latissimus dorsi. Now here's the tricky part, Dr. Westcott says, switch hands and brush your teeth with your left hand. Then put your right arm over your head and stretch to your left. You can repeat these stretches two or three times.

BONUS: Your teeth should be very clean!

Part 4

NUTRITION
NEWS

CHAPTER 14

TEST YOUR NUTRITION IQ

Take our quiz and then learn the latest strategies to make a good diet great

You're no slouch: You know a calorie from a carbohydrate and consider nutrition labels required reading. But are you eating the right foods to help you lose weight, build bone, and protect your heart? Answer the following questions to see if you're making the best choices to safeguard your health for life.

Q: *You're stuck in a breakfast meeting and starving. Which would be the lowest-calorie choice from the tray of baked goodies?*

    A. Blueberry muffin

    B. Butter croissant

    C. Cinnamon chip scone

ANSWER: B. All that air inside makes the sinful-sounding croissant (about 355 calories) much less calorie-dense than the scone (470) or muffin (500). If you're trying to lose weight, capping breakfast at about 400 calories is smart.

    Even smarter would be bringing a healthy snack to munch on during mealtime meetings, such as peanut butter on whole wheat or a bag of nuts and dry whole grain cereal.

Q: *Now that manufacturers have filtered trans fats out of many foods, they are replacing partially hydrogenated oils with other types. Which of these should you be avoiding, too?*

A. Soybean oil

B. Palm oil

C. Corn oil

ANSWER: B. Tropical oils—such as palm and coconut—are usually solid at room temperature, so they give products about the same shelf life that trans fats provide. That's great for food makers, not so great for your heart: Palm oil is 51 percent saturated fat, coconut oil more than 90 percent. Just like trans fats, saturated fat boosts levels of "bad" cholesterol and raises your risk of heart disease.

Scan ingredient lists for liquid olive or canola oils instead; they're low in saturated fat and high in heart-healthy monounsaturated fat. Nonhydrogenated corn, soybean, and safflower oils also make good trans-free substitutes.

Q: *True or false: "Organic" and "natural" on a label mean basically the same thing.*

ANSWER: False. For a label to earn a USDA-certified organic seal, it must meet specific government standards. Organic meat, poultry, and dairy come from animals that aren't given hormones or antibiotics, and organic crops are grown without using most conventional fertilizers, synthetic pesticides, or bioengineering. Natural, on the other hand, is loosely defined as not containing synthetic preservatives or artificial color or flavor; the term is not regulated.

Though many foods labeled natural are healthy, some, like all-natural soda and chips, are still loaded with calories and sugar.

Q: *You need potassium to keep your metabolism revved and muscles strong. Which of these offers the most?*

A. One medium baked sweet potato

B. One cup of fat-free yogurt

C. One medium banana

ANSWER: A. It contains 542 milligrams; the yogurt has 475 milligrams and the banana, 422 milligrams. Other potassium-rich foods to help you reach the recommended 4,700 milligrams per day (amounts listed in milligrams per cup): tomato sauce (811), orange juice (496), and cantaloupe (427).

Q: *Which ground meat makes the healthiest low-fat burger?*

    A. Ground beef
    B. Ground turkey
    C. Ground chicken

ANSWER: They all can (if you choose wisely). For ground beef, look for 90 to 95 percent lean on the label, which equates to less than 10 grams of fat per 3.5-ounce serving. Just a few percentage points lower can make a big difference: 85 percent lean beef packs a whopping 18 grams of fat per serving, which is about the same as a McDonald's Quarter Pounder.

With turkey and chicken, ground breast is better than regular (because the high-fat skin doesn't get processed in), and extra-lean is best, with less than 5 grams of fat per serving.

Q: *Of these fast-food sandwiches, which has more calories than a McDonald's Big Mac?*

    A. Wendy's Chicken Club
    B. Arby's Roast Turkey & Swiss
    C. McDonald's Premium Grilled Chicken Classic

ANSWER: B. Sure, it sounds healthy, but with its supersize slabs of bread, you get 725 calories, 8 grams of saturated fat, and more than a full day's worth of sodium! Order it without the mayo to make it healthier, and then save half for the next day.

Q: *If you must have chips, which of these is the most nutritious?*

    A. Banana chips
    B. Veggie chips
    C. Potato chips

ANSWER: B. Veggie chips made from real vegetables are the best of the bunch—with only about 150 calories per serving. (Some not-so-healthy varieties contain mostly flour and food coloring, so check the ingredient list.) Potato chips take a surprise second, with the same calories per handful as veggie chips and lots of choices with little (or no) saturated or trans fats. Banana chips should be skipped altogether: A serving is loaded with 10 grams of fat, nearly all of which is saturated.

Q: *Lose 5 pounds in 3 months if you skip your daily dose of this popular coffee-shop drink:*

A. Small cappuccino
B. Small light Frappuccino
C. Small vanilla latte

ANSWER: C. At 190 calories, a vanilla latte is heftier than the cappuccino or light Frappuccino (about 90 calories each). Skim 60 calories off your latte by requesting fat-free milk and just two pumps of syrup.

For more tricks to cut 100 calories, visit prevention.com/100calories.

Q: *Calcium is key to building bones, but which of these dairy foods is not a good source?*

A. Cottage cheese
B. Yogurt smoothie
C. Fat-free milk

ANSWER: A. The combination of low calories and high protein makes cottage cheese the perfect waist-friendly food. But during processing, up to 75 percent of the calcium drains away, leaving each $\frac{1}{2}$-cup serving with only 70 milligrams of calcium—less than half of what you get in the same amount of fat-free milk.

To meet your daily calcium needs (1,000 milligrams for age 50 and younger; 1,200 milligrams for age 51 and older), choose foods with 20 to 30 percent of the daily value (200 to 300 milligrams) listed on the label.

Q: *Which salty snack contains the most sodium?*

A. One sourdough pretzel

B. 17 salt-and-vinegar potato chips

C. A quarter cup of salted peanuts

ANSWER: A. Just one sourdough pretzel tips the sodium scale at 500 milligrams; eat three and you've hit your limit for the day if you're over age 50. (The chips have 380 milligrams, and the nuts only 115 milligrams.)

A food is considered low sodium if it contains 140 milligrams or less per serving. If you have slightly elevated blood pressure, pay close attention to sodium counts: Cutting back may lower your risk of cardiovascular disease by up to 25 percent, according to a recent study published in the *British Medical Journal*.

Q: *Which of these salad toppings will set you back the most calories?*

A. Roasted almonds

B. Butter-garlic croutons

C. Crispy chicken

ANSWER: C. Tossing in a few crispy chicken strips adds 330 calories and 17 grams of fat. Opt for grilled chicken (at only 150 calories and 4 grams of fat) and pile on mandarin oranges and cherry tomatoes (for delicious and nutritious added volume and vitamins).

Enjoy ¼ cup of nuts on occasion. Although they're high in calories, they offer good-for-you fats. But skip the croutons and crispy noodles altogether because they're just empty calories.

Find ways to make more of your favorite meals healthier at prevention. com/mealbalancer.

Q: *Which of these swaps is worth making?*

A. Brown sugar for white

B. Sea salt for table salt

C. Light olive oil for regular

ANSWER: None of them!

Where to look on a food label, whether you want to protect your heart, lose weight, or build bone

How often do you look at the nutrition facts on the products you buy?

If you said frequently, you're being smart about your health. Adults who read food labels slash twice as many calories from fat as those who don't give them a look, according to a study published in the *Journal of the American Dietetic Association*. But that doesn't mean you have to read every line, every time you shop.

Whether you want to gain energy, protect your heart, lose weight, or more, you can make the best choices for your objective by scanning a few select pieces of information. Here's where to look depending on your health goal, plus the spot that deserves a second glance.

To Gain Energy

FOCUS ON WHOLE GRAINS. Scan the ingredients list for the word *whole* before grains such as wheat, corn, barley, rye, and rice. (Millet, amaranth, quinoa, and oats are whole grains, too.)

Whole grains sustain energy because they keep blood sugar stable. Refined carbohydrates (such as white sugar and flour) cause big spikes and drops in sugar levels that can leave you feeling drained, says Tara Gidus, RD, a spokesperson for the American Dietetic Association.

Daily goal: At least three 1-ounce servings of whole grains

GLANCE AT IRON. Look for 10 percent Daily Value (1.8 milligrams) or more in each serving.

Without enough iron in your blood, your cells don't get the oxygen they need, and that causes fatigue, says Nancy Clark, RD, author of *Nancy Clark's Sports Nutrition Guidebook*. It's especially important to add iron-enriched packaged foods to your diet if you don't eat red meat.

Daily goal: 18 milligrams for women age 50 and younger; 8 milligrams for women age 51 and older

To Lower Cholesterol

FOCUS ON SATURATED FAT. Look for 1 gram or less per 100 calories. (If the food has 200 calories per serving, it should have no more than 2 grams of saturated fat.)

Most of the cholesterol in your blood doesn't come from high-cholesterol foods; it's actually made by your body, and the culprit is saturated fat. The more you consume, the more cholesterol your body makes. So even if you see *cholesterol free* stamped on the package, the food may still be a bad choice if it's loaded with saturated fat.

Of course, you can still indulge in a little saturated fat-filled ice cream or cheese now and then. You just have to plan for it. A ½-cup scoop of your favorite flavor, for example, may have 13 grams! Save it for a splurge and shoot for a minimal amount of sat fat the rest of the day.

Daily goal: No more than 10 percent of your daily calories. (For a 1,600-calorie day, that's 17.5 grams of saturated fat.)

GLANCE AT TRANS FAT. Look for 0 grams in the nutrition facts and no hydrogenated anything in the ingredients list.

Trans-free products are easier to find these days, but manufacturers can still claim "no trans fats" if there's less than 0.5 gram per serving. Eat two servings, and you may get nearly 1 gram of trans fat. That's enough to raise your "bad" LDL cholesterol and, worse, reduce your "good" HDL cholesterol. That's why you have to scan the ingredients list, too.

"Don't eat it if you see the word 'hydrogenated,'" says David L. Katz, MD, MPH, director of the Yale Prevention Research Center in New Haven, Connecticut. "Look for trans-free products that list liquid canola and olive oils instead."

Daily goal: As close to 0 grams as possible

To Preserve Memory

FOCUS ON OMEGA-3S. Look for it touted on the food package, not on the label.

A slew of products, including cereal, eggs, and juice, are fortified with omega-3 fatty acids, but you won't find any values for them listed on the product nutrition label. Instead, a statement, usually found on the front of the package, will say how much of this fat the food contains.

(continued)

A study done at the Rush Institute for Healthy Aging in Chicago showed that older adults who got omega-3s from at least one fish meal a week were 60 percent less likely to develop Alzheimer's disease than those who rarely or never ate fish.

Daily goal: 1,000 milligrams

GLANCE AT TOTAL FAT. Make sure most (about three-quarters) is poly- and/or monounsaturated fat. (If a food has 10 grams of total fat, 7 to 8 grams of it should be unsaturated.)

Foods that are high in polyunsaturated and monounsaturated fats (such as oils and margarines, for example) list both values on their labels. Just add them up to see if they equal about three-quarters of the total fat count. (If the label only lists saturated fat and trans fats, subtract them from the total fat count to get an unsaturated count.)

It's worth the effort: Researchers at the Rush Institute also discovered that unsaturated fats may defend against Alzheimer's disease. People who ate about 24 grams of monounsaturated fat per day had an 80 percent lower risk of disease than those who got only 15 grams, they found. A diet that's higher in unsaturated fats improves your cholesterol profile, and that can help keep brain cells healthy, too.

Daily goal: Total fat less than 30 percent of your daily calories, with about three-quarters of that coming from unsaturated fat

To Lose Weight

FOCUS ON CALORIES. Look for low counts and large servings.

It's the golden rule: Take in 500 fewer calories each day, and you drop 1 pound per week. So looking for low-cal meals and snacks makes sense.

But when you're standing in the supermarket reading the back of a snack-size box of raisins, for example, how do you know if 130 calories is too high or low? The key is to compare similar types of food and pay attention to serving sizes. You get 1.5 ounces of raisins for those 130 calories, but a pineapple snack bowl offers 4 ounces of fruit for only 54 calories.

Considering the servings per container helps keep you on track, too: Most soup brands contain two servings per can, so double the calorie count if you normally eat an entire can in one sitting. The same goes for beverages: A 20-ounce soda bottle contains 2½ servings; at 100 calories per serving, you consume 250 if you drink the whole thing.

Daily goal: About 1,350 calories per day if you are average height and not very active; up to 1,800 if you are tall or if you exercise three or more times per week

GLANCE AT FIBER. Look for 3 to 5 grams per serving.

High-fiber foods help you stay slim because they fill you up with fewer calories and slow down digestion so you feel fuller, longer. An analysis of research published in *Nutrition Reviews* showed that people who added 14 grams of fiber to their diet more than 2 days a week lost about 1 pound a month.

Daily goal: At least 25 grams

To Strengthen Bones

FOCUS ON CALCIUM. Look for 20 to 30 percent Daily Value (200 to 300 milligrams) per serving.

Adding calcium-rich foods to your diet is better than simply relying on supplements, says Robert P. Heaney, MD, a professor of medicine at Creighton University Medical Center. The interaction of nutrients, such as protein and magnesium, helps your body use the calcium better. And postmenopausal women who get most of their calcium from foods have higher bone density than those who just pop calcium pills, says a new study published in the *American Journal of Clinical Nutrition*.

Daily goal: 1,000 milligrams for women age 50 and younger; 1,200 milligrams for women age 51 and older

GLANCE AT VITAMIN D. Look for at least 10 percent Daily Value per serving. (That equals 40 international units, or IU.)

Typically, only foods that are fortified with vitamin D—such as milk, some ready-to-eat breakfast cereals, and orange juice—have it listed on the food label. (Natural sources include wild-caught salmon, sardines, and whole eggs.) This vitamin helps transport calcium from the digestive tract into your blood. Without D, your body might only absorb up to 10 percent of dietary calcium.

Daily goal: 400 to 800 IU for women age 49 and younger; 800 to 1,000 IU for women age 50 and older

CHAPTER 15

Be a Savvy SHOPPER

Simple, smart ways to stock your pantry and refrigerator with healthy foods and make it easier to eat well

If your kitchen is stocked with chips and dips, no wonder it's going to your hips! On the other hand, eating well is easy if you have plenty of healthy foods that are easy to eat. Here's how to set yourself up for success.

HEALTH SURPRISES IN YOUR PANTRY

Cutting your grocery bill is no reason to sacrifice flavor or nutrition. Stock your kitchen cabinets with low-cost health superstars—such as canned and jarred beans—so you always have a good-for-you meal at your fingertips. Bonus: These foods don't spoil as quickly as fresh. Here are five cupboard staples we love—and simple steps to transform them into quick meals.

Chickpeas: In a recent study, adults who ate 3 cups of chickpeas—aka garbanzo beans—a week cut both total and bad cholesterol by 7 points.

Try: Crunchy chickpeas: Rinse and dry chickpeas, spray lightly with oil and spices, and bake until golden brown.

Canned wild salmon: It contains heart-healthy omega-3 fatty acids and fewer pollutants, like PCBs, than farmed.

Try: Light salmon salad: Blend salmon with olive oil, lemon juice, dill, and capers and use in sandwiches and salads.

Artichoke hearts: They have inulin, which is a prebiotic fiber that boosts gut health and may even help control appetite.

Try: Mediterranean artichoke omelet: Sauté garlic, drained artichokes, and spinach for a delicious, nutritious omelet filling; top with crumbled feta and oregano.

Diced fire-roasted tomatoes: Processed tomatoes are richer in the skin-protecting antioxidant lycopene than fresh.

Try: Pasta with a kick: Sauté onion, red-pepper flakes, garlic, tomatoes, oregano, parsley, and basil; toss with whole grain penne.

Beets: The antioxidant betanin may prevent cancer and heart disease.

Try: Beet, walnut, and greens salad: Top baby arugula with beet slices; sprinkle with goat cheese, walnuts, and balsamic vinaigrette.

SMART BUYS AT THE HEALTH FOOD STORE

Health food stores are booming: 469 new establishments opened between 2005 and 2006, for a total of 35,876 nationwide. Unfortunately, many shoppers believe that everything they sell is healthy—and that the staff is knowledgeable about nutrition. Neither is necessarily true.

It's not uncommon for the staff's "nutrition smarts" to come from popular bestsellers and word-of-mouth advice. Some of the information is valid, but not all. Here are the top lessons we wish everyone knew.

Don't be fooled by fat fads. Bad fats are unhealthy by any name. Ghee (clarified butter), promoted as a healing food in Ayurvedic medicine, doesn't deserve a health halo. It contains the same amount of artery-clogging saturated fat as does regular butter, and four separate studies found it to promote cardiovascular disease.

Also, beware of artisan cheeses and premium ice creams. They're high in saturated fat and calories. Stick with liquid vegetable oils, trans-free spreads, and low-fat cheeses, all found in abundance at these stores.

Stock up in the dairy section. It's a dietitian's dream, overflowing with healthy dairy and nondairy selections, which makes it easy to get the bone-building calcium you need. The options are amazing: low-fat, creamy Greek-style yogurt made from sheep's or goat's milk; kefir and other products with friendly bacteria that improve digestive health and boost immunity; plus soy- or rice-based items that are low in saturated fat, says Susan Moores, RD, a Minnesota-based spokesperson for the American Dietetic Association (ADA).

Don't assume that the hot food bar is healthier. Freshly made doesn't necessarily mean good for you. For example, mashed potatoes prepared with butter, whole milk, and salt, and bakery goods made with eggs, butter, and cream are fresh and unprocessed, but they can be high in saturated fat, cholesterol, and sodium per serving. Organic macaroni and cheese can range upward of 410 calories and 16 grams of fat.

Instead, load up on healthy salad bar items, including marinated vegetable and whole grain salads, olives, and cooked beans. Homemade soups such as Tomato and Garden Vegetable, Chicken Noodle, and Carrot Ginger from Wild Oats are all 120 calories or less per cup.

On the hot bar, avoid creamy sauces. Instead look for potatoes with skins, and choose dishes with colorful fruits and vegetables as the predominant ingredients, recommends Moores.

Check out the faux meats. Health food stores are one of the few places that carry an extensive variety of "vegetarian meats," including ready-to-eat, high-protein, fiber-rich, cholesterol- and saturated-fat-free lunchmeats, hot dogs, burgers, and sausages. Incorporating more vegetarian proteins into your diet and eating less saturated fat helps reduce the risk of developing heart disease.

You can find a meat-free version of just about everything, including pepperoni, bacon, even chorizo. Choosing veggie chorizo saves 7 grams of saturated fat, compared with the real thing, and adds 6 grams of fiber for double the portion.

Don't get your vegetables in the supplement aisle. Most natural food emporiums have sizable supplement departments, compared with supermarkets, accounting for up to 15 percent of the square footage of some stores. Though supplements can help round out nutritional shortfalls, they can't replace the thousands of natural nutrients in whole foods.

"Never spend more on supplements than you do on food," says Dawn Jackson Blatner, RD, a spokesperson for the ADA. "Healthy food does a much better job of meeting your body's wide-ranging nutrient needs for much less money."

Look for local produce. A health food store can be the next best thing to a farmers' market. Whole Foods, for example, aims to dedicate 20 percent of its produce section to locally grown fruits and veggies. Buying local has its advantages: Because the distance from the farm to your plate is shorter, it's good for the planet because fewer carbon emissions are created in transit. Plus the food is more nutrient packed than varieties from distant lands. Pennsylvania State University scientists discovered that even when spinach was properly stored, it lost nearly 50 percent of its nutrients in 8 days' time.

But aside from nutrition, local produce is simply fresher and tastier, says Marion Nestle, PhD, MPH, a professor of nutrition, food studies, and public health at New York University and author of *What to Eat*. That means you're more likely to eat several servings by day's end rather than tossing out limp, tasteless produce you never touched.

Don't fall for "natural sugar" traps. It's true that "healthy" snack foods don't contain high fructose corn syrup or white sugar, but they can still be loaded with sugars in disguise, such as turbinado, sucanat, and Florida sugar crystals. The latter are derived from sugarcane or beets, which are the same sources for refined sugars.

Dr. Nestle points out that these foods are just as high in calories without any added nutrition value. And they can be much more expensive. For example, all-natural Sundrops provide more calories and cholesterol per gram than their classic counterpart, M&M's. An oatmeal-raisin cookie by Alternative Baking Company, Inc., is cholesterol and egg free and made with organic unrefined cane sugar, but it still contains a whopping 480 calories and 18 grams of fat.

Instead, buy cookies sweetened with fruit juice that are lower in fat, such as Fabe's brand, which have 90 calories and only 4 grams of fat per serving (3 very small chocolate chip cookies). Choose oatmeal-raisin or peanut butter varieties for an extra nutrition kick. If portion control is a problem, buy one fresh bakery cookie instead of a box.

Gobble up the whole grains. Whole grain products are typically plentiful at these stores, including 100 percent whole grain burger and hot dog buns, crackers, cereals, pitas, and pastas. These selections make it easy to feed your kids whole grain versions of the foods they love, such as pizza or mac 'n cheese.

The stores also stock many frozen whole grain items, such as waffles, pancakes, pizza crusts, and meals—like Ethnic Gourmet Chicken Biryani over Brown Rice or Amy's Breakfast Burrito made with a whole grain tortilla.

Don't take advice from the clerk. Employees are not required to complete any formal education or training in nutrition science. That means you might know as much as they do about what to eat and why. Even worse, they could give you advice that harms rather than helps.

If you're looking for a registered dietitian for one-on-one advice, find one in your zip code at eatright.org.

Take a lesson. Many health and natural food stores schedule specialty classes not typically offered by mainstream markets, such as RD-led nutrition seminars and healthy cooking demos. Check with your local stores.

GREAT NUTRITION ON ICE

A lot of people think fresh is best, but believe it or not, frozen produce is even more nutrient packed. That's because the moment produce is picked, it starts to lose nutrients, but freezing slows that loss. A 2007 study found that the vitamin C content of fresh broccoli plummeted 56 percent in 7 days, but it dipped just 10 percent in a *year*'s time when frozen at −4°F (−20°C). In addition, the levels of disease-fighting antioxidants called anthocyanins and some minerals, including potassium (which helps control blood pressure), actually *increased* after freezing.

According to the CDC, you should be eating about 2 cups of fruit and 2½ cups of veggies each day. (One cup is about the size of a baseball.) Fortunately, hitting the mark is easier than you may think. Just 12 frozen baby carrots equal a cup, and with no washing or chopping required, your veggies are ready in no time. From freezer to fork, most veggie side dishes take less than 10 minutes. Here's how to select and prepare 'em.

Pick US Grade A. For quality, generic is just as good as name brands, if you choose US Grade A (also known as Fancy) varieties. This ranking means the produce was carefully selected for color and tenderness and is free from blemishes. It'll be more flavorful, compared with Grade B (also called Extra Standard), which is slightly more mature, or C (Standard), which is not uniform in color or flavor.

Grade C veggies are the least expensive, and though they still provide nutrients, they can be stringy, tough, even bitter. It's best to use them in recipes that don't feature them prominently, such as soups, stews, and casseroles. Grades usually appear on the back of the package, inside a symbol that looks like a shield.

Skip added sauces. When sauces and seasonings are included, fat, sodium, and sugar levels typically skyrocket. The healthiest choices are bags and boxes with zero additives. That means selecting products with only vegetables listed in the ingredients. Many shoppers think frozen goods are heavily processed. They can be, but not in this case. Freezing itself is enough to preserve produce without the addition of salts (which can raise blood pressure) or sugars (which spike blood sugar).

Though some manufacturers claim their sauce is light or low fat, that doesn't mean it's healthy. A 10-ounce package of broccoli in low-fat white Cheddar cheese sauce provides nearly 15 times as much sodium as an entire 12-ounce bag of plain broccoli florets. A 16-ounce package of strawberries in sauce contains 285 more calories and an additional 77 grams of sugar, compared with a 20-ounce bag of frozen whole strawberries; that's nearly 20 teaspoons' worth.

Bottom line: Eating frozen produce in sauces is definitely better than eating none, but we strongly recommend sticking with unseasoned vegetables, especially because you can easily (and healthfully) dress them yourself.

Add flavor without lots of calories. Pick the right topping, and you can have low-cal, low-sodium veggie side dishes in minutes. Just add jarred vegetable tapenades or pestos. They are rich in flavor and coat vegetables perfectly, and most add a mere 40 calories and almost no sodium. Microwave or steam your favorite frozen vegetable, and toss with 1 tablespoon per cup of vegetables. Here are our favorite combos.

- Sun-dried tomato pesto with cut broccoli florets or spinach
- Olive pesto with green beans
- Artichoke tapenade with yellow wax beans
- Wild mushroom pesto with Brussels sprouts
- Butternut pesto with carrots
- Ginger glaze with Oriental veggies or shelled edamame

CHAPTER 16

Pick More
PRODUCE

*Get everyone to eat more greens—and reds
and oranges—with these novel strategies*

VEGGIES, FAMILY STYLE

Once, your kids loved vegetables, but then they stopped thinking it was fun to stick peas up their nose. Now, chances are, they're like most Americans—falling woefully short of the three to eight servings of vegetables that nutritionists say they should eat each day. You're probably not doing much better: Most adults don't even manage to hit the old five-a-day goal.

Think veggies take too long to cook? Find them bitter or boring? We took five of America's favorite vegetables and made them tastier and a snap to prepare.

Potatoes

Spuds with skin are packed with vitamin C and are one of the best sources of potassium and fiber. They can be low cal: A plain baked potato has only 140 calories. Trouble is, we love to fry them or load them with sour cream, butter, or gravy. Here's how to make them healthy.

Veggie baked potato: Scoop out the flesh of a baked potato and mash with steamed broccoli and 1 percent cottage cheese to add protein and calcium (but few calories). Stuff the filling back into the skin.

Mayo-free potato salad: Toss steamed, quartered new potatoes with steamed green beans; add honey mustard mixed with a bit of olive oil to make an easy side dish.

Pasta, potato-style: Pick up some gnocchi (a pasta made from potatoes) in the refrigerated section of the grocery store. Cook according to the package instructions and add pesto sauce and steamed peas. A serving of gnocchi contains about 4 ounces of potatoes.

Or try cauliflower instead. It's a natural substitute for potatoes because it shares the same hearty texture. Nuke and puree it and use as a creamy base for soup, or coat florets with olive oil and curry powder and roast them.

PREVENTION
Alert!
⟶
....

THE ORGANIC ADVANTAGE

Compelling new research from the United Kingdom finds more proof that organics are better for you. When farmers grew produce on adjacent organic and conventional farms across Europe, the organic fruits and vegetables had up to 40 percent more disease-fighting antioxidants than the conventional produce. For example, researchers found that organic apples had a 34 percent increase in antioxidant activity versus conventional ones. Also, milk from cows raised organically contained up to 80 percent more of the healthful compounds than milk from traditionally raised cattle.

Here's a fast way to find organic produce at the grocery store: Look at those pesky stickers. A 4-digit number means the food was conventionally grown; a 5-digit number beginning with 9 means it was grown organically.

"If you buy a conventional banana at the grocery store, the sticker will read 4011. An organic one will say 94011," says Barbara Haumann, spokesperson for the Organic Trade Association. Our recommendation: Check for the 9 on produce you eat most often.

Carrots

These crunchy root veggies are vitamin A powerhouses, but they're typically served raw or steamed—in other words, bland and uninspired. Here's how to make them tasty.

Power sandwich: Spread whole wheat bread with peanut butter, and top it with raisins and shredded carrots for an interesting crunch, great taste, and a hint of sweetness.

Honey carrots: Boil baby carrots until just tender. Add a dab of butter and honey to make a kid-pleasing classic.

Low-fat fries: Using regular or multicolored carrots (available in red, white, yellow, and purple at natural food stores), slice lengthwise and coat with olive oil, salt, and pepper. Roast in a 425°F oven for 30 to 40 minutes.

Or try butternut squash instead. Like carrots, this yellow-orange veggie becomes sweeter when cooked. Roast and toss in soups, pastas, and stews. Or puree it and season with cinnamon and maple syrup for a delicious side.

Tomatoes

Tomatoes are our most common source of lycopene, which is an antioxidant that might protect against heart disease and breast cancer. But we generally eat them in the form of sugar-loaded jarred spaghetti sauce or use only a thin slice in a sandwich. Here's how to make tomatoes dazzling.

Tomato tower: Stack slices of tomatoes with thin slices of fresh mozzarella and fresh basil. Drizzle with extra virgin olive oil and balsamic vinegar. Try orange tomatoes, found in gourmet grocery stores: Their lycopene is more easily absorbed than the red variety's.

Roasted tomato–topped chicken: Quarter plum tomatoes and coat with olive oil, garlic powder, salt, and pepper. Roast in a 400°F oven for 20 minutes. Serve over grilled chicken breasts.

Southwestern rice: Toss canned diced tomatoes and mild canned chile peppers with instant brown rice, and cook. Add shredded cheese.

Or try red bell peppers instead. One bell pepper packs more than 100 percent of your daily dose of vitamin C; in texture and color, the red or orange varieties are good tomato alternates. Roast and puree for a tangy pasta sauce, stuff with sautéed ground turkey and bake, or sub slices for chips with dip.

Broccoli

The antioxidants in this vegetable may prevent colon and lung cancer, and its calcium is more easily absorbed than the calcium from milk, so it's a natural bone builder. But we usually serve this veggie raw (a major turnoff for most kids) or, even worse, overcooked to an unappetizing olive hue. Here's how to make it kid friendly.

Guilt-free dips: Microwave broccoli florets and cool. Serve it with low-fat ranch dressing or a protein-rich hummus for adults or kids with more sophisticated tastes.

Pasta primavera: Mix microwaved florets with cooked penne pasta, sautéed chicken tenders, marinara sauce, and a dash of red-pepper flakes.

Super salad: Microwave florets and cool. Combine with halved grape tomatoes, lemon juice, and olive oil. The healthy fat helps your body absorb more vitamins.

Or try asparagus instead. This broccoli cousin is milder and more pleasant to young palates. Buy several bunches, coat with olive oil, and roast. Leftovers are great hot or cold, and you can use them in pastas, sandwiches, and salads.

Corn

This whole grain is rich in fiber (1 cup provides nearly 5 grams), and it contains antioxidants that promote eye health. Unfortunately, we keep serving it the same old way: boiled and boring or slathered in butter. Here's how to make corn festive, even fun.

Polenta parmigiana: Cook polenta (made from cornmeal, a more concentrated source of nutrients than fresh corn) according to package directions. Top with marinara sauce and low-fat mozzarella.

Spicy chicken salad: Combine canned black beans, corn kernels, roast chicken, and scallions. Dress with olive oil, a squeeze of lime, and a dash of chili powder.

Creamy corn: Mix equal parts frozen corn and canned creamed corn, which is naturally low in fat but has a consistency kids love. Warm it over medium heat and sprinkle with shredded low-fat cheese.

Or try peas instead. A member of the legume family, peas trump corn in both protein and fiber. Make an easy hummus with frozen baby peas: Cook 1 cup and then puree in a food processor with olive oil and lemon juice. Season

---

EAT-SMART TIP

Skip iceberg. It's relatively low in nutrients. Instead, hit up a salad bar at a gourmet grocery store or deli and combine antioxidant-packed varieties such as arugula, watercress, mustard greens, spinach, and radicchio.

with salt, pepper, and garlic powder. Or add peas to rice for a hit of color—and a more filling side dish.

THE VEGETABLE GENIUS

For even more ways to make inspired vegetables, we went to the expert. For more than three decades, Mollie Katzen has been transforming the humble veggie into something extraordinary. Here's how she does it—and how you can, too.

"Don't they look just delicious?"

Mollie Katzen is standing before a crowd of foodies, holding a plate of simply prepared green beans. Their vibrant color jumps off the plate, and the air is filled with the bold, spicy scent of fresh garlic. All the food lovers in attendance draw a little closer, hoping to catch a whiff and, if they're lucky, a free sample. They know: If anyone can make a plate of veggies worthy of such desire, it's Katzen.

Katzen might not have a cooking show or a magazine bearing her name, but to many healthy cooks—not to mention some of the country's most esteemed dietitians and public health experts—she is nothing less than an icon. She made a national name for herself as the Julia Child of vegetarian cuisine when Ten Speed Press published her first book, *Moosewood Cookbook*, in 1977, and *Enchanted Broccoli Forest* in 1982. But these days, she shuns the label.

"Vegetarianism is perceived as being about restricting certain foods, and that's not what I'm all about," she says. "I want people to eat vegetables because they're some of the tastiest foods in the world."

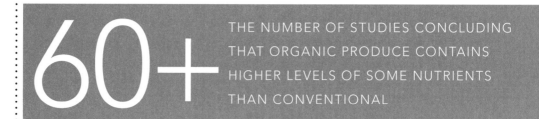

60+ THE NUMBER OF STUDIES CONCLUDING THAT ORGANIC PRODUCE CONTAINS HIGHER LEVELS OF SOME NUTRIENTS THAN CONVENTIONAL

SMALL FRUIT, BIG BENEFITS

When it comes to produce, smaller may be superior nutritionally. As fruits and vegetables grow larger, their vitamins, minerals, and other health-boosting compounds significantly diminish, according to a recent report issued by the Organic Center, a nonprofit organization that gathers science on the health benefits of organics. Taste and aroma decrease as well.

Although the losses occur in organically grown produce as well as conventional, organic items tend to be smaller in general—making shopping those aisles a simple way to maximize your nutrient intake.

It's Katzen's reputation for creating mouthwatering plant-based meals that has made her the go-to chef for such healthy eating experts as Walter Willett, MD, DrPH, chair of Harvard University's nutrition department. In 1998, Dr. Willett invited Katzen to join the Harvard Nutrition Roundtable, which is a think tank of sorts where researchers present their latest findings to a select group of food professionals. Back then, Dr. Willett's team was turning up groundbreaking science on the benefits of diets containing healthy fats and whole grains, but they needed someone to take the message public. Katzen was a natural choice.

"She's not just interested in nutrition science, but highly skilled at translating research into recipes," says Dr. Willett.

Over the past decade, their collaboration has extended beyond the Roundtable to other projects, including the book *Eat, Drink, and Weigh Less.* "In Mollie's hands," he says, "a vegetable is a starting point that turns out to be infinitely variable and interesting. The journey can be spectacular."

For Katzen, her role as the missing link between nutrition science and culinary art is a comfortable fit. "My goal is to completely erase the line in the sand between what's healthful and what's delicious," she says. By following these five strategies, inspired by the recipes in Katzen's latest book, *The Vegetable Dishes I Can't Live Without,* you, too, can watch that line disappear.

Be Open

One of the simplest ways to eat healthy is to, as Katzen says, flip the plate paradigm: Think of vegetables as the main attraction with protein in the supporting role. Be open to the idea that vegetables really are appealing enough to take the lead. These meaty mushrooms, for instance, are hearty enough to satisfy even a meat lover.

PORTOBELLO PARMESAN

MAKES 4 SERVINGS

Portobello mushrooms are one of the best sources of selenium, which may help protect against cancer. Adequate selenium is also required for DNA repair.

1 tablespoon extra virgin olive oil

4 firm portobello mushrooms (4" diameter), stems and gills removed (leave edges of caps intact)

¾ cup fat-free ricotta cheese

½ cup shredded reduced-fat mozzarella cheese

1 large clove garlic, minced (1 teaspoon)

Ground black pepper

1 medium firm-ripe tomato, thinly sliced

1 tablespoon fresh thyme leaves

3 tablespoons grated Parmesan cheese

1. **PLACE** a large ovenproof skillet over medium heat. After about a minute, add the oil and swirl to coat pan. Lay the mushrooms cap-side down in skillet and cook undisturbed about 10 minutes. Turn and cook on the other side for 10 minutes. Turn over again.

2. **COMBINE** the ricotta, mozzarella, and garlic in a small bowl. Season with the freshly ground black pepper to taste.

3. **SPOON** about 3 tablespoons of the ricotta mixture into each mushroom cap (leave in the pan), spreading gently into place.

4. **PREHEAT** the broiler.

5. **ARRANGE** a few tomato slices on each mushroom and sprinkle evenly with the thyme and Parmesan. Broil about 5 minutes or until the tops turn golden brown. (Watch carefully to prevent burning.)

NUTRITIONAL INFO PER SERVING: 156 calories, 12 g protein, 11 g carbohydrates, 2 g fiber, 7 g fat, 2.5 g saturated fat, 214 mg sodium

Be Quick

Like most of us, Katzen has little time to think about dinner, so she often relies on quick-cooking techniques to coax the most flavor out of veggies in the shortest amount of time. In this recipe, for example, green beans are sautéed quickly over high heat, giving them a rich, savory flavor. You can use the same cooking method with virtually any vegetable that's cut into thin strips, so they heat through quickly. Try it with a mixture of fennel and bell peppers another time.

DRAMATICALLY SEARED GREEN BEANS

MAKES 4 SERVINGS

This method works best when the beans are as fresh as possible—straight from the farmers' market if you can swing it. Bonus: The fresher the bean, the more nutrients it packs.

2 tablespoons canola or peanut oil

1 pound whole green beans, trimmed

2 large cloves garlic, minced (1 tablespoon)

⅛–¼ teaspoon red-pepper flakes

1. **PLACE** a large, deep skillet or wok over medium heat. After about 2 minutes, add the oil and swirl to coat the pan.

2. **RAISE** the heat to high and wait about 30 seconds. Add the green beans and season with salt to taste. Cook for 3 minutes, shaking the pan and/or using tongs to turn and move the beans so they cook quickly and evenly. Carefully taste the beans (may be crunchy) and cook until the desired doneness.

3. **SEASON** with the garlic and red-pepper flakes to taste. Cook for 1 minute longer. Serve hot, warm, or at room temperature.

NUTRITIONAL INFO PER SERVING: 98 calories, 2 g protein, 8 g carbohydrates, 4 g fiber, 7 g fat, 0.5 g saturated fat, 7 mg sodium

Be Creative

The artist in Katzen (she began her culinary career as a way to support her art studies) loves to play up the natural beauty of fresh fruits and vegetables—one reason her recipes have instant appeal to a wide audience. Think of vegetables as a palette of colors and textures that can be combined and composed artfully on the plate, such as this salad.

BEET-AVOCADO-PEAR "CARPACCIO"

MAKES 6 SERVINGS

Arugula is an excellent bone builder, supplying vitamin K, calcium, and magnesium. If you find its flavor too strong, try sweet-tasting baby arugula.

2 cups arugula leaves

2 packages (8 ounces each) cooked, drained, peeled red or golden beets, thinly sliced

1 tablespoon roasted walnut oil

1 medium avocado, halved, pitted, peeled, and thinly sliced lengthwise

1 tablespoon cider vinegar

2 medium pears, thinly sliced

1 tablespoon freshly squeezed lemon juice (½ lemon)

¼ cup crumbled Roquefort or Gorgonzola cheese (1 ounce)

¼ cup finely chopped walnuts, lightly toasted

1. SCATTER the arugula onto medium-large serving platter or on 6 small plates. Arrange the beets on the plate and drizzle them with the oil. Arrange the avocado on the plate and immediately drizzle with the vinegar to keep from discoloring. Sprinkle with salt to taste.

2. LAY the pear slices on the plate and sprinkle the entire salad with the lemon juice. Toss the cheese over top and sprinkle with the walnuts.

NUTRITIONAL INFO PER SERVING: 191 calories, 4 g protein, 20 g carbohydrates, 6 g fiber, 12 g fat, 2 g saturated fat, 149 mg sodium

Be Bold

Part of what gives veggies such versatility in Katzen's hands is the way she uses techniques and ingredients from other cultures. If you've only known eggplant in eggplant Parmesan, for instance, you might not recognize it in this dish. Katzen takes advantage of the vegetable's absorptive qualities to soak up a sauce that captures the hot, spicy, salty, and sweet flavors of Thailand. It's literally a world away from eggplant Parm.

SOUTHEAST-ASIAN-STYLE EGGPLANT

MAKES 4 SERVINGS

Eggplant notoriously absorbs a lot of oil, so don't be tempted to add more. If you need more liquid for cooking, simply splash in a bit of water.

2 tablespoons canola or peanut oil

2 large eggplants (about 3 pound), peeled and sliced lengthwise (½" thick) and then crosswise into ½"-thick sticks

1 medium red onion, sliced (1 cup)

¼ teaspoon salt

3 large cloves garlic, minced (2 tablespoon)

3 serrano chile peppers, thinly sliced (use plastic gloves when handling; avoid touching eyes)

⅓ cup dry sherry or ¼ cup rice wine vinegar

¼ cup water

2 tablespoons packed brown sugar

2 tablespoons reduced-sodium soy sauce

2 tablespoons freshly squeezed lime juice (1 lime)

1 cup (packed) fresh mint leaves, coarsely chopped

1. PLACE a large skillet or wok over medium heat. Swirl in the oil to coat the pan. Add the eggplant, onion, and salt and cook, stirring, about 5 minutes.

2. ADD the garlic, peppers, and sherry and cook, stirring, for 5 minutes longer.

3. COMBINE the water, sugar, soy sauce, and lime juice in a small bowl and stir until the sugar dissolves. Stir into the eggplant mixture. Cover, reduce the heat to low, and cook, stirring frequently, for 10 minutes or until the eggplant has reduced in volume by about half.

4. REMOVE from the heat and stir in the mint.

NUTRITIONAL INFO PER SERVING: 212 calories, 5 g protein, 33 g carbohydrates, 13 g fiber, 8 g fat, 0.5 g saturated fat, 428 mg sodium

Be Playful

Katzen's sense of humor and joy plays a huge role in her approach to food. Her book *Enchanted Broccoli Forest* was named after the "broccoli trees" that poked out of an herbed rice pilaf recipe. The point? Don't be afraid to have fun with your food, as with these cucumber boats. And the next time you make a rice pilaf, go ahead, plant a few broccoli trees.

FETA-WALNUT STUFFED CUCUMBERS

MAKES 4 SERVINGS

Salty feta mixes nicely with the flavor of slightly bitter walnuts, a prime source of omega-3 fats, which may enhance brain function.

½ cup walnut halves

¼ cup chopped fresh parsley

½ cup crumbled feta cheese (about 2 ounces)

¼ cup fat-free milk

1 small clove garlic, minced (½ teaspoon)

½ teaspoon mild ground paprika

⅛ teaspoon ground red pepper

4 medium cucumbers, peeled, halved lengthwise, and seeded

1. **COMBINE** the walnuts and parsley in a blender or food processor and pulse until powdery in texture. Add the cheese, milk, garlic, paprika, and ground red pepper and puree until smooth.

2. **FILL** the cucumbers with the feta-walnut mixture, patting into place with the fork or spoon. Slice into wedges and lightly sprinkle the tops with a little extra paprika.

NUTRITIONAL INFO PER SERVING: 164 calories, 6 g protein, 8 g carbohydrates, 3 g fiber, 12.5 g fat, 3.5 g saturated fat, 222 mg sodium

DELICIOUS CITRUS

Even when the weather outside is frightful, in the produce aisle a rainbow of yellows, oranges, pinks, and greens lights the way. Citrus fruits are nature's gift to winter: colorful, sweet, and packed with immune-boosting nutrients, right smack in the middle of sick season.

For years, dietitians have championed the health benefits of these fruits' star vitamin: C. Although getting enough C won't prevent you from catching a cold or flu, studies show that it could help you recover faster.

"Normal blood levels of vitamin C are absolutely critical for optimal immunity," says Simin Nikbin Meydani, DVM, PhD, a professor of nutrition and immunology at the Friedman School of Nutrition Science and Policy and Sackler Graduate School at Tufts University. And new research conducted at Purdue University has revealed that the C in citrus juices may boost your body's absorption of the cancer-fighting compounds in tea.

But bear in mind: Your body doesn't store vitamin C, so you need to replenish your supply every day. You'll get a day's worth in one orange or grapefruit, 6 ounces of orange juice, or two clementines.

Shopping tip: Search for extra-heavy fruits. More weight means more juice and additional nutrients. Then, eat them out of hand or prepare one of the following delicious desserts, each of which supplies a serving of sunshiny citrus goodness.

PREVENTION Alert!

THE POWER OF THE PEEL

When you squeeze a lemon (or peel an orange), save the skin. Scientists at De Montfort University in the United Kingdom found that a compound in tangerine peel called salvestrol Q40 kills an enzyme that spurs the growth of human cancer cells. Previous research has shown that limonene, a compound found in lemon, orange, and grapefruit peel, might also decrease cancer risk. Zest the well-washed fruit (toss the bitter white pith) and add to soups, baked goods, yogurt, or hot tea.

TANGELO TIRAMISU

Like clementines, tangelos are virtually seedless, making them a great snacking fruit. A tangelo is a hybrid of a grapefruit and a tangerine. Minneola, a popular variety, has deep red-orange skin and a knobby projection at the stem end; one fruit also fulfills an impressive 80 percent of your daily folate need. In the kitchen, a small, serrated knife is the best tool for peeling and sectioning the fruit.

6 Minneola tangelos (2¼ pounds)

⅓ cup sugar

⅓ cup fat-free cream cheese, softened

¼ cup mascarpone cheese

1 package (3 ounces) ladyfingers (about 12)

1. **REMOVE** the peel and white pith from the tangelos and cut the sections from the membranes. Place the sections in a medium bowl. Squeeze the juice from the membranes into a small bowl.

2. **BEAT** the sugar, cream cheese, and mascarpone until smooth in a medium bowl.

3. **SPLIT** the ladyfingers lengthwise in half. Pour half of the tangelo juice into a pie plate or shallow dish. Dip the flat sides of half of the ladyfingers into the juice. Arrange flat-side-up in 8" x 8" baking dish. Spread half of the cheese mixture over top and cover with half of the tangelo sections. Repeat with the remaining juice, ladyfingers (place flat-side-down on fruit), cheese mixture, and fruit. Cover with plastic wrap and chill for 2 to 24 hours to allow the flavors to blend.

NUTRITIONAL INFO PER SERVING: 237 calories, 6 g protein, 35 g carbohydrates, 3 g fiber, 10.5 g fat, 5 g saturated fat, 101 mg sodium

23

THE PERCENTAGE OF FRUIT IN THE UNITED STATES THAT GOES TO WASTE, ACCORDING TO THE USDA

CLEMENTINE AND GRAPEFRUIT COMPOTE

MAKES 4 SERVINGS

Clementines are a type of mandarin orange. Virtually seedless and supereasy to peel, they're perfect when you're on the go. Two fruits pack a day's worth of vitamin C for just 70 calories. Here, they're paired with ultrahealthy grapefruit in a refreshing compote that can be served as a dessert, salad, or sweet salsa.

4 clementines

2 grapefruits

Grated zest of 1 lime

3 tablespoons honey

1. REMOVE the peel and white pith from the clementines and grapefruits and cut the sections from the membranes into a large bowl. Squeeze the juice from the membranes over fruit. Add the lime zest and honey and mix gently.

2. SERVE in small cups or bowls and top with additional lime zest, if desired.

NUTRITIONAL INFO PER SERVING: 143 calories, 2 g protein, 38 g carbohydrates, 7 g fiber, 0.5 g fat, 0 g saturated fat, 1 mg sodium

1
THE AMOUNT OF CALORIES FOUND IN A TEASPOON OF LEMON ZEST, ACCORDING TO THE USDA

HOW TO BUY, STORE, AND SERVE CITRUS FRUIT

Fruit is delicious and nutritious—nature's perfect snack food. Here's how to enjoy it—effortlessly.

BLOOD ORANGE: The bright red flesh signals the presence of disease-fighting anthocyanins.

Tastes: Sweet and tart with a hint of raspberry

Storage tip: Keep oranges away from foods that absorb odors, such as eggs and cheese.

CLEMENTINE: At 35 calories each, these are a nutritional bargain.

Tastes: Tangy-sweet

Buying tip: Clementines are often sold in crates; look through the bottom slats to spy any damaged specimens.

GRAPEFRUIT: Red grapefruit might help lower levels of LDL cholesterol, according to research published in the *Journal of Agricultural and Food Chemistry*. But beware: Grapefruit juice should not be consumed with several prescription drugs, including cholesterol-lowering statins.

Tastes: Bittersweet

Buying tip: Skin should feel springy yet firm.

KEY LIME: This citrus is brimming with phytochemicals, such as hesperidin, which may protect against cancer.

Tastes: Sweet-tart

Storage tip: Humidity keeps limes juicy; store in a plastic bag in the refrigerator for up to 10 days.

KUMQUAT: Four walnut-size kumquats offer 5 grams of heart-helping fiber, which is more than a fifth of the daily value.

Tastes: Sweet peel and tart flesh (Eat the whole thing!)

Storage tip: Wrap in a plastic bag and refrigerate up to 2 weeks.

MEYER LEMON: The zest is also a good source of limonene, which is an antioxidant compound that might help prevent cancer.

Tastes: Sweet and tangerine-like (best for desserts)

Serving tip: Use this extra-sweet lemon for pies, lemonade, and other treats.

NAVEL ORANGE: This winter stalwart is known for its high vitamin C content; one fruit supplies 110 percent of the Daily Value.

Tastes: Sweet and juicy

Buying tip: Green skin isn't a sign that it's underripe.

POMELO/PUMMELO: One half of a pomelo is a good source of fiber, supplying 3 grams.

Tastes: Varies from tangy-tart to spicy-sweet

Serving tip: The pomelo is related to the grapefruit and can be substituted for it in recipes.

SOUR ORANGE: One orange contains 29 percent of the recommended daily intake of vitamin A.

Tastes: Bitter and acidic

Serving tip: Use the juice (often sold bottled) in marinades for pork or seafood.

TANGELO: One fruit delivers 4 percent of the Daily Value of calcium.

Tastes: Sweet-tart and juicy

Serving tip: Pair with crisp fruits, such as apples and pears, in a salad for a megadose of vitamins.

TANGERINE: Supplies thiamin, which is a B vitamin that your body needs to produce energy from carbohydrates.

Tastes: Juicy and subtly tart

Serving tip: Stir fruit into yogurt or use its juice in dressings or marinades.

ORANGE AND PEAR CRISP

MAKES 8 SERVINGS

Eating sweet oranges—one of the most popular fruits in the world—might lower your risk of rheumatoid arthritis, ulcers, and lung cancer. Oranges contain an anti-inflammatory compound called hesperidin, which lab studies indicate may help lower cholesterol.

½ cup all-purpose flour

¼ cup + 2 tablespoons granulated sugar, divided

¼ cup packed brown sugar

¼ cup cold trans-free margarine, cut into small pieces

8 medium seedless (navel) oranges

2 large pears (1 pound), peeled, cored, and cut into 1½"–2" chunks

1 tablespoon cornstarch

¼ teaspoon freshly grated nutmeg

1. **PREHEAT** the oven to 400°F.

2. **COMBINE** the flour, ¼ cup of the granulated sugar, and brown sugar in food processor. Add the margarine and process until crumbly.

3. **REMOVE** the peel and white pith from the oranges and cut the sections from the membranes into a large bowl. Squeeze juice from membranes over fruit. Add the pears, cornstarch, nutmeg, and remaining 2 tablespoons sugar. Mix gently. Spoon into eight 6-ounce ramekins or an 8" x 8" baking pan. Sprinkle with the flour mixture. Bake the individual ramekins for 15 minutes and the square pan for 30 minutes or until golden brown.

NUTRITIONAL INFO PER SERVING: 227 calories, 2 g protein, 46 g carbohydrates, 5 g fiber, 4.5 g fat, 0.5 g saturated fat, 46 mg sodium

MAKES 4 SERVINGS

Pink and red grapefruits get their hues from lycopene, which is one of the most potent anti-cancer carotenoids. Adding a rich pomegranate syrup—packed with anthocyanins—gives an extra health boost.

1 cup pomegranate juice

¼ cup + 2 tablespoons sugar, divided

2 red grapefruits, peeled (white pith removed) and each cut into 4–6 round slices

1. **COMBINE** the juice and ¼ cup of the sugar in a small saucepan. Bring to a boil, reduce the heat, and simmer, stirring occasionally, for 20 to 25 minutes or until reduced to ⅓ cup. Cool to room temperature.

2. **PREHEAT** the broiler with the rack about 4" from the heat.

3. **ARRANGE** the grapefruit slices in a single layer in a large baking dish. Sprinkle with the remaining 2 tablespoons sugar. Broil for 6 minutes or until the grapefruit is flecked with brown. Arrange on serving platter or individual plates and drizzle with the pomegranate syrup.

NUTRITIONAL INFO PER SERVING: 144 calories, 1 g protein, 37 g carbohydrates, 1 g fiber, 0.5 g fat, 0 g saturated fat, 8 mg sodium

PREVENTION Alert!

THE RIPE FRUIT ADVANTAGE

If those pears seem a little overripe, don't toss 'em. Fruit at or just past its peak contains disease-fighting antioxidants called nonfluorescing chlorophyll catabolites, according to a study from the University of Innsbruck in Austria. A recent Belgian study found that overripe produce is packed with other healthful compounds, even if it doesn't look picture-perfect.

To disguise bruises: Cut into chunks and simmer with a bit of water into a sauce, or blend with ice for a smoothie.

CHAPTER 17

Health Food IMPOSTORS

Some foods that have an undeserved reputation as virtuous choices—and here's the new research on what you should eat instead

Even if you haven't bought full-fat mayo or sugary soda since blue eye shadow was in style (the first time), you may be getting duped into less-than-stellar food choices at the supermarket. The culprit? The "health halo."

"From a distance, some foods seem like healthful choices because of the way they're packaged or labeled," says Janel Ovrut, MS, RD, a Boston-based dietitian. "But just because a product's marketing gives it an aura of health doesn't necessarily mean it's good for you." Here are eight notorious health food impostors, plus smarter swaps that up the nutritional ante and still give you the flavor you crave.

IMPOSTOR: BAKED POTATO CHIPS

Yes, they're lower in fat. But they're still high in calories and low in nutrients, with little fiber to fill you up.

Smarter sub: Popcorn. You'll get the salt and crunch of chips plus fiber, and around 65 percent fewer calories per cup. Look for oil-free microwave popcorn or brands that are air-popped or popped in healthful oils such as olive or canola.

Health bonus: Heart-healthy whole grains. Adults who eat popcorn take in as much as 2½ times more whole grains than people who do not, according to a recent study published in the *Journal of the American Dietetic Association*.

Try: Good Health Half Naked pre-popped popcorn, made with olive oil. One serving (4 cups) has 120 calories, 0 grams sat fat, and 4 grams fiber.

IMPOSTOR: GUMMY FRUIT SNACKS

Although these products may contain some juice, they're usually nothing more than candy infused with some vitamins. They also contain high fructose corn syrup, which is linked with obesity, and they have heart-unhealthy partially hydrogenated oils.

Smarter sub: Fresh or dried fruit. Both are packed with filling fiber, which you'll miss if you opt for gummy snacks.

Health bonus: Cancer-fighting antioxidants. Real fruit is loaded with immune-boosting nutrients that fruit-flavored snacks could never mimic. A

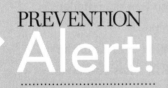

PREVENTION Alert!

AMERICA'S HEALTHIEST MUSHROOM

Ironically enough button mushrooms have a terrible, and undeserved, reputation with most folks. They're not colorful, but mushrooms have a brilliant reputation with dietitians. Tufts University researchers found that white buttons ward off viruses and tumors in mice by boosting the immune system's killer cell activity. They might protect against cancer, thanks to potent antioxidant levels.

Added bonus: Cup for cup, swapping rice or spaghetti for mushrooms can save up to 200 calories. (Try it. We swear you'll like it.) Do that twice a week, and you can drop 6 pounds in a year.

recent Greek study found that women who ate the most fruits and veggies were the least likely to develop any type of cancer.

Try: Peeled Snacks Fruit Picks dried fruit (peeledsnacks.com). One serving (one bag) of Go-Mango-Man-Go has 120 calories, 0 grams sat fat, and 2 grams fiber.

IMPOSTOR: LIGHT ICE CREAM

Light ice cream can have fewer calories than regular, but there's no guarantee. Take Häagen-Dazs Dulce de Leche light ice cream: With 220 calories per ½ cup serving, it's still higher in calories than the average full-fat ice cream, which has around 140 calories per serving. What's more, some light ice creams can lack the rich taste you crave, so you're less satisfied and may be inclined to eat more than one serving.

Smarter sub: Dairy-free ice cream. Soy and coconut milk ice creams may save you a few calories, and they have a creamy, satisfying texture.

Health bonus: Digestion-friendly fiber. Some dairy-free ice creams are made with chicory root, a natural source of inulin, a prebiotic fiber that can increase healthy bacteria in the gut and help the body absorb calcium and iron.

Try: Turtle Mountain Purely Decadent, made with coconut milk. One serving (½ cup) of vanilla has 150 calories, 7 grams sat fat, and 6 grams fiber. (Studies show that the saturated fat in coconut might not raise cholesterol like the saturated fat in butter and meat.)

IMPOSTOR: DIET SODA

In a 2008 study, researchers linked drinking just one diet soda a day with metabolic syndrome, which is the collection of symptoms including belly fat that puts you at high risk of heart disease. The researchers aren't sure if it's an ingredient in diet soda or if it's the drinkers' eating habits that caused the association.

Smarter sub: Flavored seltzer water. It has zero calories and is free of artificial sweeteners but provides fizz and flavor. Beware of clear sparkling beverages that look like seltzer yet contain artificial sweeteners. They're no better than diet soda. Or try a sparkling juice; we recommend watering it down with seltzer to stretch your calories even further.

Health bonus: Hydration without chemicals. Water is essential for nearly every body process.

Try: Your supermarket's low-cost seltzer brand. The taste is the same as the bigger name brands.

IMPOSTOR: "CALORIE-FREE" SPRAY MARGARINE

Even though some spray margarines claim to be "calorie-free," labeling laws allow products with fewer than 5 calories per serving to claim to have zero calories. So, while one spritz may be inconsequential, the whole bottle could have as much as 900 calories.

Smarter sub: Spray-it-yourself olive oil. In this case, a bit of real fat is more healthful and flavorful—and within a reasonable calorie range if you watch your portions. Investing in an olive oil mister ensures you don't put on too much.

Health bonus: Decreased inflammation throughout the body, which helps your heart and lowers cancer risk, thanks to monounsaturated fatty acids.

Try: Misto olive oil sprayer. Buy one at any kitchen store for around $10.

IMPOSTOR: NONFAT SALAD DRESSING

Fat-free salad dressings are often packed with sugar—so your dressing may be loaded with calories. Ironically, a salad without fat is not living up to its potential. "You need a little fat to absorb vitamins A, D, E, and K and other nutrients," says Katherine Tallmadge, RD, spokesperson for the American Dietetic Association.

Smarter sub: Oil-based salad dressings. You'll get good-for-you fats instead of the saturated fat found in some creamy dressings. Look for ingredients like olive oil, vinegar, and herbs.

Health bonus: Vision protection. As many as five times more carotenoids—antioxidants that are essential for eyesight—are absorbed when salads are consumed with fat rather than with no fat.

Try: Newman's Own Olive Oil & Vinegar Dressing. Two tablespoons have 150 calories, 2.5 grams sat fat, 0 grams fiber.

IMPOSTOR: LOW-FAT COOKIES

Do you remember the SnackWell's craze? Low-fat cookies are still popular, and many dieters think they can indulge guilt free. The problem is that most

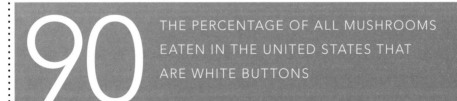

90 THE PERCENTAGE OF ALL MUSHROOMS EATEN IN THE UNITED STATES THAT ARE WHITE BUTTONS

of these snacks are made with extra sugar, which means they often have just as many calories as the full-fat version, if not more.

Smarter sub: Oatmeal cookies. These are a great way to indulge a cookie craving while also getting whole grains. Not all are created equal, though: Skip those made with high fructose corn syrup, white flour, and butter in favor of varieties made with honey or cane juice, whole wheat flour, and oil.

Health bonus: Lower cholesterol. The fiber found in oatmeal keeps your body from absorbing bad cholesterol.

Try: Kashi TLC Cookies. One cookie has 130 calories, 1.5 grams sat fat, 4 grams fiber.

IMPOSTOR: 100-CALORIE SNACK PACKS

You might want to skip these if you're trying to lose weight. A recent study showed that people may eat more food and calories if the portions are presented in small sizes and packages. With smaller serving sizes, study participants didn't feel the need to regulate their intake, so they ate more than one portion before feeling satisfied.

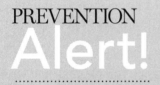

PREVENTION Alert!

SNACK SMARTLY

Are you unconsciously overeating foods that you think are healthful? When Cornell University professors hosted a group of movie watchers, they gave each guest a bag of low-fat granola. Half the group's granola was labeled low-fat, while the other half's was marked regular. By the flick's end, the low-fat group had eaten 50 percent more than those who thought they were eating regular—a total of 249 calories, the amount found in a glazed doughnut.

Plan ahead. Keep calories from snacks in check: Portion 150 to 200 calories' worth into a ziplock bag or bowl.

Smarter sub: A small serving of almonds. Their healthy monounsaturated fat, fiber, and protein will tide you over until your next meal.

Health bonus: Stronger bones. Almonds are an excellent source of bone-building magnesium, as well as the immune-boosting antioxidant vitamin E.

Try: Blue Diamond Natural Oven Roasted Almonds. A 1-ounce serving has 160 calories, 1 gram sat fat, 3 grams fiber.

Spot a health fraud! You can learn more good and bad nutrition picks at prevention.com/impostors.

CHAPTER 18

Give Your WATER a Makeover

Flavored waters are a great way to meet your hydration needs, but some have as much sugar as a can of soda. Here's smart new advice on how to sip right

Most of us are lousy at drinking water. We'll drink coffee and tea till the cows come home, but we have to force down plain water because it's just so, well, plain.

Don't feel guilty, though. Humans and animals alike are pretty picky about fluids. We prefer them flavored, and we drink more when the taste is appealing. These inherent preferences probably have a lot to do with the incredible surge of bottled waters, with newfangled flavors such as jasmine vanilla and raspberry cream. During a recent grocery trip, we counted no less than 20 different brands. The food industry even has a name for them: New Age beverages. The category also includes natural sodas, herbal teas, smoothies, and other drinks sought out by those of us looking for a healthier substitute.

Soda sales recently dropped for the first time in 35 years, and flavored water purchases have grown 36 percent since 2005. Although some really are healthful, others are merely glorified soft drinks.

TESTING THE WATERS

So how do you make the best choice for your waistline—and your health? Several flavored waters simply offer a tastier way to stay hydrated. Others contain additives such as vitamins, antioxidants, herbs, and caffeine, and make claims about helping you relax, boosting your energy level, and supporting your immune system. And though they're called water (which we think of as calorie free), some have as many calories as a snack—and cost nearly as much as a barista-made latte.

But flavored water's newfound popularity is encouraging, because water is the single most important nutrient for your body, regulating temperature and filtering out waste, and it makes up 60 percent of your weight. Ready to take the flavored plunge? Here's our three-step plan for healthfully navigating the sea of options.

AVOID SUGAR AND ARTIFICIAL SWEETENERS

Flavored waters are typically sweetened with natural sugarcane or fructose (fruit sugar) rather than high fructose corn syrup, the sweetener found in soda

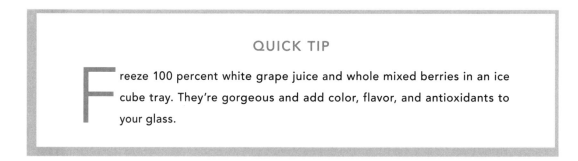

QUICK TIP

Freeze 100 percent white grape juice and whole mixed berries in an ice cube tray. They're gorgeous and add color, flavor, and antioxidants to your glass.

that's linked to obesity and type 2 diabetes. But some 16-ounce bottles provide as many as 180 calories, just 20 shy of a same-size Coca-Cola Classic.

That's important because research shows that caloric beverages aren't filling. When Purdue University scientists fed two groups the same number of calories from either soda or jelly beans for 28 days, the candy group naturally compensated by eating less food—while the soda group did not. In the end, the jellybean eaters' weights stayed the same, but the soda group gained weight. If you don't burn it off, a bottle-a-day habit can add 19 pounds to your frame over a year.

And artificial sweeteners aren't the solution. When researchers at the University of Texas Health Science Center at San Antonio followed more than 1,000 people for 8 years, they found that on average, for each diet soft drink consumed per day, the chances of becoming overweight or obese jumped about 37 percent. This is probably due to an interesting phenomenon other studies have found: Even "fake" sugars increase the preference for sweets.

KEEP IT NATURAL

We think of water as pure, but even waters that seem wholesome can be loaded with artificial colors, flavors, and preservatives. (We call them "Twinkie" waters.) Look beyond the label and check the ingredient list.

You might see plenty of words more reminiscent of a chemistry lab than a mountain spring, such as sodium hexametaphosphate (a flavor protector also used in ceramics), sodium benzoate (a preservative and precursor to benzene, acknowledged by the FDA as a known cancer-causing substance), and ETDA (a stabilizer used in laundry detergents). Only buy brands that have terms you recognize.

A CLEAR LOOK AT WATER BOTTLES

A *Prevention* reader asks, "Should I stop using plastic water bottles?" The short answer is no. You don't need to round up your plastic water bottles and banish them to the recycling bin. But reducing their use—drastically, if possible—is a smart idea for your wallet, the environment, and your health.

We've fielded lots of questions on this topic lately. A favorite came from a 9-year-old girl participating in one of our studies on environmental contaminants, who asked: "What's the problem, anyway? I'm not eating the bottle, just drinking the water." Putting the smarty-pants factor aside, it's a good point. But chemicals from the plastic end up in the water, and scientists are trying to figure out whether this should worry us. In a report released last April, the federal government's National Toxicology Program expressed "some concern" that one chemical in many plastics could harm children's neurological development and reproductive organs.

The possible bad guy is a chemical called bisphenol A, also called BPA. Increasingly strong evidence suggests that BPA is an endocrine disruptor, which means it can mimic or block the function of hormones. In animal research, BPA and other endocrine disruptors have been linked to a range of unwanted effects—earlier puberty in females, enlarged prostates in males, and even cancer. (One recent review suggested that in some circumstances, endocrine disruptors could increase the risk of obesity!)

BPA is in many sports bottles, watercooler jugs, and baby bottles. These are usually marked by a "7" inside the recycling symbol (though not all "7" products contain BPA). Heating these bottles can be particularly problematic: When scientists

BEWARE OF HEALTH PROMISES

You've probably seen flavored waters that promise to calm you or boost energy. They are typically fortified with vitamins, minerals, caffeine, and herbs like passionflower. But some don't have studies to back their claims. One supposed metabolism-boosting water, for example, offers no published studies using the water itself, nor is there evidence that the key ingredient is effective for weight

poured boiling water into a number 7 plastic bottle, BPA entered into the water 55 times faster than when they used water at room temperature. So don't put your sports bottle (or a baby bottle!) into the dishwasher or microwave.

On the other hand, you may be relieved to hear that most of the single-serving water bottles sold at grocery stores don't contain BPA. They're made of polyethylene terephthalate (PETE or PET), designated by a number "1" in the recycling sign. But even though PETE doesn't contain BPA, it does contain other chemicals called phthalates, which are also believed to be endocrine disruptors. Like BPA, these chemicals leach into the water more quickly when the plastic is heated, so don't leave these water bottles in a hot car or out in the sun.

This isn't a panic situation. But you get BPA and phthalates from many sources in the environment—so why increase your consumption if you can avoid it? Get cheaper, greener, and healthier water by taking the following easy steps.

AT HOME: Save yourself some money—and save the environment some grief—by drinking from the sink. Municipal tap water is constantly tested to ensure its safety. If you don't like the chlorine taste or are concerned about other impurities such as lead, use an activated carbon–based filter. Brita and PUR are popular brands, and both companies say that their plastic pitchers contain no BPA.

ON THE GO: Put your tap water into an aluminum or stainless steel sports bottle, such as those by Klean Kanteen or SIGG—or a new, BPA-free plastic sports bottle from Nalgene.

IN A STORE: For those parched times when you don't have your own bottle handy, pick bottled water instead of a sugary drink. Just be sure to recycle!

JAZZ UP PLAIN WATER

For a cheaper—and just as tasty—alternative to flavored waters, try these do-it-yourself tips.

Tangy: Squeeze in wedges of lemon, lime, tangerine, or pink grapefruit, or mix water with unsweetened infused herbal-flavored tea.

Sweet: Chill with cubes made from 100 percent juice, bits of real fruit, citrus zest, and spices, or add a splash of 100 percent juice such as white grape or apple.

Spicy: Stir in fresh mint, lemongrass, or grated ginger.

loss. Also, waters that are heavily fortified with vitamins and minerals may actually suppress your immune system if your combined vitamin/mineral intake from food and these waters boosts you over acceptable limits.

Bottom line: Don't look to waters to meet nutrient needs or provide benefits above and beyond hydration. Water itself is pretty great on its own!

SOUND ADVICE

THE THREE BEST NUTRITION CHANGES TO MAKE TODAY

We asked James O. Hill, PhD, director of the Center for Human Nutrition and a professor of pediatrics and medicine at the University of Colorado Health Sciences Center, what are the top three nutrition changes to make to boost your health. Without a moment's hesitation, here's what he advised.

1. STOP EATING JUST A LITTLE BIT EARLIER. By the time your body tells you that you're full, most people have eaten too much, says Dr. Hill. We're not talking about depriving yourself, he adds. Just stop eating a little bit before you clean your plate. Wait a few minutes, and then your natural satiety cues will kick in and tell you that you're full. That way you can avoid eating too much, and that feeling that you're too full.

2. DRINK WATER. We've gotten away from drinking water as a beverage, Dr. Hill says. Yet, natural, plain water is the beverage we should be drinking. When you drink beverages other than water, you're likely drinking far too many calories. Rediscover water instead.

3. GET A PEDOMETER. While this might seem like an unusual suggestion for a nutritional change, here's why it works. If you take more steps, it gives you more wriggle room in your diet, Dr. Hill says. For less than $20, you get a tool that will help you to be more active. Keep track of how many steps you take each day, and simply try to go up a little each day. That'll allow you to put more fun into your diet.

Part 5

MIND
MATTERS

CHAPTER 19

BOOST YOUR BRAINPOWER

Here's how to never forget anything (anymore)

Four superbusy women boost their brainpower with the help of memory makeovers from the nation's top brain experts.

GOAL: "HELP ME PREVENT ALZHEIMER'S"
TERESA MCCOART, 51, SENIOR ADMINISTRATIVE ASSISTANT

"I watched both my parents lose their memories, so I'm taking steps to help protect mine—starting today," Teresa says.

The expert: Vincent Fortanasce, MD, a Neurological Rehabilitation Specialist at the Fortanasce Neurology Center in Acadia, California

When Teresa forgets the names of her coworkers, she isn't just embarrassed, she's scared. Before her parents passed away, they both developed dementia, which is a disorder that impaired their memory, judgment, and motor skills. (The most common causes are Alzheimer's and stroke.) Teresa was concerned that her "senior moments" were signs she'd suffer the same fate.

If Teresa were to inherit the disease, she would develop symptoms when her parents did. (They were in their 70s.) Instead, Dr. Fortanasce believes her poor lifestyle habits are to blame for her blank moments now, though they might put her at a higher risk for memory loss later. The good news: There's still plenty of time to make adjustments.

"Genes determine 30 percent of your risk of developing Alzheimer's," says Dr. Fortanasce. "The other 70 percent comes from factors you can control—diet, fitness, and stress levels." Though Teresa did recently start exercising, which has been shown to help slow mental decline, she should also make the following changes.

Eat more brain food. Dr. Fortanasce recommended she add 1 cup of blueberries to her daily diet. Studies show that they contain compounds that improve short-term memory. She should also increase her intake of fruits, vegetables, and fatty fish (such as salmon) to help protect and nourish brain cells; cut saturated fat to keep her heart strong and pumping blood to her head; and replace refined grains with whole ones to keep brain fuel reserves full.

Sleep 8 hours every night. Your brain needs sleep to function properly: It uses the "downtime" to sort and store information. Plus, new research suggests sleep helps strengthen memory recall. To help Teresa get more than her regular 5 hours, Dr. Fortanasce suggested she cut down on fluids and keep her bedroom cool (around 63°F), quiet, and dark.

"I sleep more soundly—and longer. I get between 7 and 8 hours now. I also made it a habit to toss blueberries in my cereal or mix them with nuts for a snack," Teresa says. "Though I still have the occasional blank moment, overall, I'm more focused, more energized, even happier. I now know how to keep my brain healthy, and I'm motivated to keep it up."

Make a brain-boosting vinaigrette. Rosemary and turmeric stimulate the brain. Dr. Fortanasce recommends adding a pinch of each, three times a day, to your food. Teresa does so by whisking them with olive oil (2 tablespoons), garlic powder (3 pinches), salt (a dash), and rice wine vinegar (to taste)—and uses the vinaigrette on salad and to marinate meat and drizzle over veggies.

GOAL: "HELP ME EXCEL AT MY NEW JOB!"
LAURIE ANDERSON, 47, TECHNOLOGY ASSISTANT

"Starting a new job with a steep learning curve made me nervous," Laurie says. To prep my brain, I played some games."

The experts: Alvaro Fernandez, cofounder of sharpbrains.com, a leading brain-fitness Web site, and Elkhonon Goldberg, PhD, Sharpbrains' chief scientific advisor and a clinical professor of neurology at New York University School of Medicine

After 10 years of teaching, Laurie decided it was time for a change. Although she was excited about her new job at a middle school, she worried that she might not be able to learn new skills fast enough.

To keep her mind fit and flexible, Laurie needs to exercise her mental muscles, says Fernandez. An active brain creates new connections between cells so it can store and retrieve information more easily. Fernandez coached Laurie through a personalized brain-fitness program; he also recommends the following.

Do something new every week. Fernandez was pleased to hear that Laurie likes to try different things because tackling unfamiliar tasks boosts short-term memory and builds up the parts of the brain that encode information.

"Just doing Sudoku or crossword puzzles, for example, is like working out your biceps but ignoring the rest of your body," says Dr. Goldberg. Instead, find about 20 minutes four times a week to do a variety of mentally stimulating activities. Switch between reading different newspapers, playing Scrabble, and learning a new function on your cell phone.

Breathe deeply. Processing new information when we're anxious is tough; the stress itself is a distraction. Fernandez taught Laurie this relaxation trick: Close your eyes, touch your pinky fingers to your thumbs, and think about that healthy feeling after a good workout. Take deep breaths and hold that thought for 30 seconds. Next, move your ring fingers to your thumbs and remember a time when you felt loved for 30 seconds. For your middle fingers, recall a caring gesture, and for your index fingers, imagine a beautiful place.

"After just a week of SharpBrains training, I surprised myself," Laurie says. "One Friday afternoon, a colleague wanted to show me a new part of the job. There were kids talking, phones ringing; it was hard to focus. I took a moment to use the relaxation technique I learned. On Monday, I was able to complete a project with no extra help."

Tease your brain. Play memory-boosting games to give your mind a workout. Laurie's favorite: a SharpBrains game based on biofeedback. As a monitor chronicled her heart rate, she played a game she could win only if she used deep breathing and visualization to lower her heart rate. Try some brainteasers at SharpBrains.com, or visit prevention.com/brainfitness for more.

GOAL: "HELP ME CLEAR MY FOGGY BRAIN"
NEERJA JAIN, 43, STORE OWNER

"I couldn't keep all my work responsibilities straight, and that put my stress level through the roof," Neerja says. "Then I learned to plan, prioritize, and even find time for me."

The expert: *Prevention* Head Coach columnist Thomas Crook, PhD, a clinical psychologist based in Florida and author of *The Memory Advantage*

Neerja owns and operates five franchised coffee stores. Between handling personnel issues, equipment troubles, budgets, and inventory—and sticking to a business plan that calls for eight more stores over the next decade—Neerja often finds herself distracted, frazzled, and anxious.

"Neerja is stuck in a vicious cycle of stress," says Dr. Crook. Studies show that oversecretion of the stress hormone cortisol inhibits brain cells' ability to communicate properly. If Neerja can't think clearly, it's harder to do her job, which causes more stress and perpetuates the cycle. Here's Dr. Crook's plan to get her back in control.

Make a list of tasks and consult it twice a day. Running from store to store and crisis to crisis while trying to keep up with her executive tasks, Neerja was asking her brain to retain too much information. She needed to get—and stay—organized so she could keep up. Dr. Crook suggested she use a handheld voice recorder equipped to hold audio files in several digital folders—one for each of her stores and one for her personal life (cost: about $100;

SWEAT AND LEARN

Exercise is the best way to improve brain health, according to John Ratey, MD, author of *Spark: The Revolutionary New Science of Exercise and the Brain.*

But the best news is you don't have to move fast to jog your memory: Italian researchers found that people age 65 and older who walked enough to burn 417 calories a week (about 5½ miles at a moderate pace) were 27 percent less likely to develop dementia than more sedentary adults. Researchers believe that the exercise may help by improving blood flow to the brain.

Go one step further and challenge your noggin to learn something new while you sweat. Here are three ways.

STUDY A LANGUAGE. Pop in a DVD and enjoy Mexico's beautiful scenery as locals teach you Spanish during your home cardio machine workout. ($49 for a set of 12; connect18.com)

TAKE A COLLEGE COURSE. Pick a passion, from science to philosophy, and sign up for a downloadable audio course taught by professors from top institutions. ($20 to $400; teach12.com)

"READ" A CLASSIC. Finally tackle *Madame Bovary* or *Crime and Punishment*—on your MP3 player, that is. There's no extra credit, except for the intellectual boost that comes with great literature. ($5 to $120; learnoutloud.com)

at most electronic stores). She should review her recorded notes at night, prioritize her to-dos, and then look over her list before work the next day. Knowing she has a plan of action will ease Neerja's anxiety, says Dr. Crook.

Schedule early morning "me" time. With Neerja's tasks mapped out and fresh in her mind, she can now use her hour-long commute to do something she enjoys: listen to music or pop in an audiobook.

"Pastimes and passions are more than indulgences. They're stress relievers," says Dr. Crook.

"I use the handheld recorder and also take notes in a little book," Neerja says. "It's amazing how such a small act made such a big difference: As soon as I stopped worrying about forgetting something, I felt calmer. Creating a

(continued on page 276)

MIRACLE-GRO FOR YOUR MIND

Prevention Head Coach columnist Thomas Crook, PhD, a clinical psychologist based in Florida and author of *The Memory Advantage* has conducted extensive research to improve our understanding of how the brain works. He is a former research program director at the National Institute of Mental Health and is CEO of Cognitive Research Corp. in St. Petersburg, Florida. Here's his easy prescription for producing new brain cells: Try something new.

In 1971, when I was 26, I bought a farm. Never mind that I had a full-time job, was finishing my PhD, and knew nothing about farming except what I read in *Mother Earth News.* But I figured out how to grow crops, fix a tractor, and raise livestock. I didn't sleep a lot, but it was exciting to be learning so much. In 1997, I bought a ranch in Zimbabwe. People thought that was strange, and it completely shook up my life, but I loved it, and it forever changed my way of looking at the world. And just this past Christmas, instead of spending the holidays with family as we've done for decades, my wife and I took a cruise to Hong Kong, Vietnam, and Thailand.

Although I undertook these adventures for many reasons, they all have one thing in common: They satisfy the brain's instinctual urge—almost like a thirst or hunger—for new experience. Animal studies have shown us that the brain rewards novelty by releasing a pleasure-inducing chemical called dopamine. Learning is reinforced because it's essential to helping the brain grow and thrive. Here's the best part: If you seek out new experiences throughout life, your brain will keep growing—sprouting new cells (neurons) and the branches between them (dendrites)—no matter your age.

Science has visual evidence of this process. Thanks to MRI technology, we can see learning centers in the human brain light up and witness the birth of neural pathways when we try something new. These signs of activity and growth are visible even in the elderly. Although you may learn new things more slowly as you get older, your capacity is largely unchanged.

What's really exciting is that new experiences needn't be dramatic or life changing to have these effects. Everyday novelty—even seemingly inconsequential acts—can benefit your brain and literally expand your mind.

So let's get started. Here are some simple ways to break routine habits that may be prematurely aging your brain. Once you understand the logic involved, you'll be able to create other little ways of introducing more novelty into your life. And just like with physical exercise, the more you can do, the more you'll benefit.

- Brush your teeth using the opposite hand.
- Reverse your usual walking, running, or biking route.
- Trade in your favorite game. If you love crosswords, do Sudoku or learn to play one of the dozens of brain-training games on your computer.
- Eat at an ethnic restaurant.
- Rearrange your furniture.
- Visit a new place this weekend, even if it's just in the next county.
- Speak to people outside your normal social circle and listen for fresh perspectives on daily life.
- Grab that recipe you clipped and head to a different grocery store to shop.

If you do even a few of these things in a single day, you'll be amazed at how all this newfound knowledge enriches your life. I may never be a great farmer, but I do have a neverending store of tips on the best ways to fix a tractor.

Craving brain food? Get a must-know factoid from *The Intellectual Devotional* delivered to your inbox weekly. Sign up at prevention.com/brainfitness.

to-do list at night helped me sleep better, too. And spending those few minutes to review my game plan before I head out to work lets me spend my morning drive catching up with friends and family on my hands-free cell."

Daydream to reduce stress. Neerja and her husband hope to open an orphanage in India, so Dr. Crook suggested she take just one moment a day to "visit" the orphanage in her mind. "It helps put everyday hassles into perspective and makes me feel more relaxed and happy," says Neerja.

GOAL: "HELP ME STAY SHARP AND FOCUSED"
RACHEL WALSH, 47, REALTOR

"I thought multitasking meant I was being more productive," Rachel says. "But I realize now the slow and steady approach is best."

The expert: Gary W. Small, MD, director of the UCLA Center on Aging and the author of *The Memory Bible*

To sell multimillion-dollar homes, Rachel needs to be fast and flexible at solving problems, closing deals, and making her clients feel that their numerous needs are her top priority. If she stumbles over a potential client's name, the person may lose confidence in her abilities.

"Rachel is a multitasker, and that keeps her attention fragmented," says Dr. Small. And as we age, changes in the frontal lobes of our brains make it

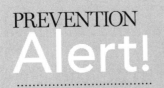

PREVENTION Alert!

NATURAL MEMORY BOOSTER
If you're feeling scattered, try caffeinated tea for a fast fix. Black, green, and oolong leaves contain the amino acid theanine, which, when paired with caffeine, boosts neural activity and concentration. For best results, combine 100 milligrams of theanine and 60 milligrams of caffeine—or 3 cups of tea, says researcher John Foxe, PhD, of the Nathan Kline Institute for Psychiatric Research in Orangeburg, New York. His tea company funded study backs up past research on theanine's mind benefits.

hard to concentrate in distracting environments. To support her memory, Rachel needs to go back to the following basics.

Take it one task at a time. Trying to do too much at once leads to forgetfulness, and Rachel often talks on the phone and reads e-mails at the same time. A mature brain tends to experience "moments of rest," resetting as we shift from one task to another, says Dr. Small. These pauses are the reason Rachel might draw a blank when she hangs up the phone or walks purposefully into a room and forgets why she needed to be there.

Say it out loud. Instead of passively taking in information, trusting that your brain will filter out the fluff while sorting and storing the important data, concentrate on being mindful. When you enter your house, for example, watch your hand place your car keys in the proper spot, even saying out loud "I'm putting the keys on their hook" to give your brain an added boost.

"My job does require some multitasking, but I make an effort to finish one thing before moving on to the next, and in the end, I'm more productive—and more organized," Rachel says. "Instead of piles of paperwork on my desk, I have bins for completed, current, and future work. This helps me look at one folder at a time."

Look, snap, connect. Dr. Small taught Rachel his all-time favorite memory-boosting trick. Here's how it works: Look reminds you to pay attention; Snap stands for taking a mental snapshot; Connect means to link the snapshot with what you need to remember. Say you meet someone named Mrs. Siegel. Look for a distinctive feature—her red hair. Picture a seagull nesting in it, and you've connected her name to her image.

Play games for healthy brains. Make your mind fit with the science-based, electronic brain games at prevention.com. Some hone memory skills, while others test language abilities. (Beware: They're addictive!) Plus, find easy de-stressing tips and exclusive memory-boosting workouts—all at prevention.com/brainfitness.

CHAPTER 20

ENERGIZE YOUR LIFE

Three exhausted women recharged their routines with simple diet, exercise, and sleep tweaks from our top medical expert. Learn how you can bust fatigue, too

Energy: You need it to exercise, to cook, to live healthy. And getting it is easier than it may seem, says Mark Liponis, MD, medical director of Canyon Ranch Health Resorts and author of *UltraLongevity: The Seven-Step Program for a Younger, Healthier You.*

"Simply shifting your thinking and making small changes to daily habits can increase your mental and physical stamina," he says. Here, he helps three women identify what's sapping their energy and offers tips on how to get it back.

If you're struggling with your own energy crisis, or even if you just need a little more pep in your step now and again, read on.

LISA ZASLOW: IN A FUNK

The less Lisa does, the less she feels like doing. As a professional organizer, she often works from home and might stay there all day. Lisa knows it's time to expand her 8-year-old business, but she feels trapped in a black hole, and she can't find the energy or motivation to pull herself out.

"I work from home, and spending most days indoors was getting me down," Lisa says. "Turns out a little fresh air can boost my mood—and energy."

Expert Advice

"Feeling blue can trigger hormonal and chemical changes that lead to exhaustion," says Dr. Liponis. Though Lisa doesn't have clinical depression, she is down in the dumps, and her environment and daily habits are largely to blame. Here are some simple tips to help brighten her mood.

Make the home office "homier." Because Lisa spends so much time in her apartment, she should feel that the space is appealing. Lisa can start by buying fresh flowers. It's not a cliché. A recent Harvard study found they help people feel happier and more enthusiastic. Also, she needs to clear piles of paper, which can be psychologically overwhelming, and hang inspirational images.

Take a breather—outside. Studies show spending time in nature can improve mood. Dr. Liponis suggests Lisa start the day with a 10-minute walk outdoors, then take at least two 5-minute walking breaks later on.

Talk to positive people. You're less likely to get depressed if you have a strong support network, according to recent research. Lisa feeds off the energy of loved ones, but her work keeps her isolated. At least twice a week, she should connect with a friend who has a healthy outlook on life.

How I Did It

"I'm a professional organizer, yet I forgot just how sensitive I am to clutter!" Lisa said. "Making my office beautiful made working at home feel like fun rather than a chore. I also try to get out and meet friends for coffee or go for a walk during the day—if not to the park, then at least around the block.

That's given me a major mental and emotional boost, and even more physical stamina: I recently had to climb six flights of stairs with a big bag of organizing supplies to a client's apartment, and I was surprised at how easily I did it."

LISA MARSHALL: BURIED BY HER SCHEDULE

As a business owner and mother of twins, Lisa has a killer routine that is jampacked and unpredictable. She's never without her laptop, squeezing in work between car pools and client meetings. As a result, she eats takeout often, barely exercises, and is constantly tired.

"My list of to-dos never ends, and I'm always tired," Lisa says. "But when I found time for me, I had more energy for everyone else."

Expert Advice

"Lisa's schedule and stress levels are so exhausting that she can't work efficiently," says Dr. Liponis. Every task takes longer to finish, leaving her no time to nurture her health. But by making self-care a priority, she'll have more energy to accomplish her to-do list. To get healthy habits into her routine, Dr. Liponis suggests the following.

Schedule workouts as appointments. A recent study found that regular exercise dramatically increased energy levels in healthy people. Lisa can combine 30 to 40 minutes of cardio 5 times a week with family time by biking with her twins, for example.

Simplify meals. Wholesome foods provide long-lasting energy, and dishes don't have to be complicated to be healthy. Lisa ought to stock up on staples that require minimal prep, such as precut veggies and frozen shrimp. Sautéed, they make a great stir-fry.

Keep a curfew. Lisa was getting between 4 and 6 hours of sleep a night; she needs 7 or 8. To get more shut-eye, she should turn off her laptop a few hours before bedtime. The light from the screen stimulates the brain, making it harder to fall asleep.

How I Did It

"Now I take a dance aerobics class that I consider mandatory, and I eat much better, especially since I discovered frozen veggies," Lisa said. "I used to think only fresh ones were healthy, but now I know that the frozen kinds have tons of nutrients and are simple, so I make them for every meal. Turning off my laptop at night has been tough, but I am trying to at least read a book before bed. I'm starting to feel good again, and people notice: After a few weeks, my friend said I seemed really 'up' about life. I couldn't believe the change was so obvious."

VERONICA EADY FAMIRA: SEDENTARY BUT TIRED

Veronica's days are always the same: She wakes up dragging, struggling to get out of bed, then spends 8 to 10 hours chained to her desk, after which she heads home to collapse on the couch and watch TV. She knows her sedentary lifestyle saps her energy, and she also knows working out would help, but she can never seem to make the effort.

"I often went from sitting at my desk to sitting on my couch at home," Veronica said. "Now I make it a point to move—even just a little—and it makes all the difference."

Expert Advice

"Veronica's right. Exercising would help her energy levels, but so would just getting up a few times during the day," says Dr. Liponis. Even three 10-minute cardio sessions every day would trigger the release of brain chemicals that increase energy. Here are Dr. Liponis's suggestions to help boost her mornings and nights.

Let in some light. Pull back the curtains first thing in the morning. Just 10 minutes of natural light is enough to alert her internal body clock that it's time to wake up.

Eat a carb-and-protein breakfast. Veronica had only coffee in the mornings, but this combination will give her body the fuel it needs to start the day

TIRED? EXERCISE ANYWAY

Step away from the remote! Ditching your workout when you're exhausted may leave you feeling worse. In a University of Georgia study, chronically tired adults who exercised at low intensity for 20 minutes 3 times a week felt 65 percent less fatigued after 6 weeks. Just keep it light. Those who stuck to low or moderate intensity also had 20 percent more energy.

and keep blood sugar even for steady energy. Try wheat toast with peanut butter, or fruit and cheese.

Limit after-work sofa sessions. Before flipping on the TV for the night, Veronica should do one thing that makes her feel "alive," says Dr. Liponis. She could volunteer at a community center, sample CDs at a music store, or browse a new art exhibit.

How I Did It

"Even on my busiest of days, I make a concerted effort to move more—just taking the stairs instead of an escalator or walking home after work," Veronica says. "Eating breakfast got me on a more regular eating schedule and gives me a little extra boost throughout the day. I'm not exactly bouncing around, but I'm definitely less tired. Plus, I had no idea that doing things after work would be so energizing: Instead of watching TV, I spend time brushing up on my German, and I'm involved with a human rights project. Now I feel engaged instead of exhausted."

THE ENERGY WORKOUT

Beat stress, boost immunity, and curb your appetite with this revitalizing 15-minute routine. With this plan, you'll gain more stamina so you can enjoy life, rather than just ending up drained and depleted. This workout features qigong, a form of active meditation, made up of flowing repetitive movements designed to harness your body's energy, which has been shown to enhance nervous system activity and lower stress hormone levels so you sleep better, feel more focused, and have fewer cravings.

A recent UCLA study found that healthy adults reported feeling 10 percent more energetic throughout the day after practicing tai chi, which is a more complex form of qigong.

A Swedish study also showed that qigong helped women in their 40s with fast-paced computer-based jobs to naturally slow their heart rate and blood pressure all day long. You can get all of these benefits and more without stressing about how to fit it in! Enter: our exclusive 15-minute routine you can do anytime, anywhere (without changing into workout clothes!). Even if you can do only a few moves a day, you'll feel happier, revitalized, and ready for your best year yet.

Taking care of ourselves right now is often last on our busy to-do list. Here are five reasons qigong is just what you need to stay healthy and happy this minute and all year long.

It brightens your mood. For adults who experience a case of the blues every now and then, doing qigong may ease depression as effectively as drugs—without the side effects—suggests a study from the Hong Kong Polytechnic University. Participants reported a 70 percent drop in symptoms after 2 months of practice, which seems to regulate serotonin levels.

It deepens your sleep. Practicing tai chi helped people with sleep complaints drift off about 18 minutes faster and slumber 48 minutes longer in an Oregon Research Institute study. The meditative movements may modify circadian rhythms, so you sleep through the night.

It revs immunity. Adults who did qigong and tai chi for 3 hours a week after receiving a flu vaccine produced three times as many antibodies as those receiving only the vaccine, reveals a study from the University of Illinois at Urbana-Champaign. This added protection could be helpful if your immune system is suppressed due to stress and lack of sleep.

It eases headaches. Qigong may also be a drug-free sigh of relief from stress-related headaches, according to UCLA researchers. Women affected by these headaches who did tai chi reported less frequent and less severe pain. The exercise limited muscle spasms and inflammation that can contribute to headaches.

It prevents slips and falls. By improving balance and reaction time, qigong can help you navigate bumpy sidewalks and slippery driveways. The slow, coordinated exercises enhance awareness of your body movement, improve control over the muscles that support the knees, and may even help you avoid a turned ankle, finds another University of Illinois study.

WORKOUT AT A GLANCE

This workout was designed by Vaishali V. Labosky, an instructor at Equinox Fitness in New York City with 20 years of experience teaching qigong and yoga. For a demo of the moves, check out prevention.com/qigong.

For all-day energy, do the routine at least 3 times a week. For an instant lift, do your favorite move anytime. Go from one exercise to the next in the order they appear, flowing through all the repetitions slowly and gracefully without stopping. Breathe through your nose, lips closed, and the tip of your tongue lightly touching the top of your mouth behind your teeth (an acupressure point thought to regulate energy).

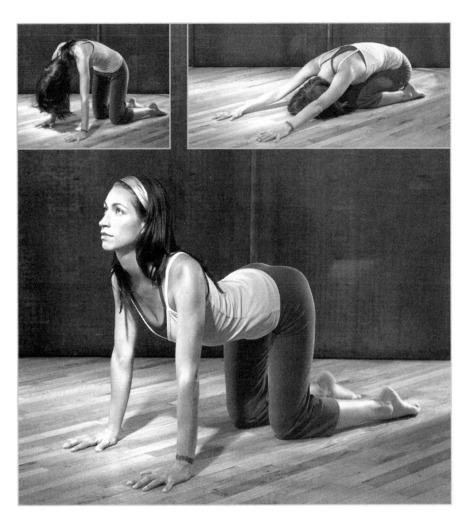

⌃ BIG CAT STRETCH

Begin on all fours, hands directly under shoulders and knees below hips, toes pointed back. Inhale, and pull belly up, rounding back toward ceiling and tucking head in to look at navel.

Exhale and sit back, reaching hips toward heels, arms extended forward.

Inhale, returning to all fours, then exhale and look upward, lifting chest and dropping belly toward floor.

For extra toning, add a yoga push-up at this point by bending elbows into sides and, on an inhale, lowering chest toward floor, keeping back curved. Exhale as you straighten arms. Repeat the sequence from the beginning. Do 3 to 6 times.

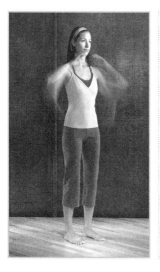

(<) HOLDING ENERGY

Come to a standing position, feet hip-width apart, knees soft, hands in front of you with elbows softly bent and pointing out to sides, palms facing up. Inhaling, slowly lift hands to chin height, then turn palms down and, exhaling, lower to hip level. Turn palms up and repeat, lifting and lowering 3 times. Turn palms to face each other, and imagine you're holding a ball. Relax eyes and focus on the space where the ball would be as you move hands slightly closer and farther apart. Notice if you feel warmth or tingling between your hands, that's your body's energy at work. Hold for about a minute.

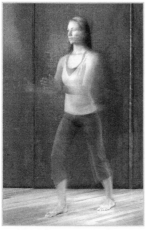

(<) ROCKING

Step right foot forward about 12 inches, arms at sides, elbows bent to 90 degrees, palms facing each other. Rock forward, bending right knee (like a lunge) as you inhale.

Extend arms upward, circling hands up and away from you. Exhale and rock back as hands circle down, bending left knee and straightening right, front foot flexed so toes are off floor. Bring hands up in front of body.

Continue rocking forward and back 6 to 9 times as you circle arms. Switch legs and repeat.

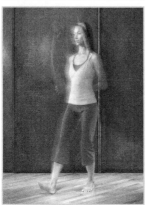

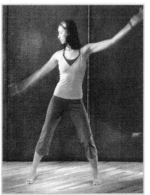

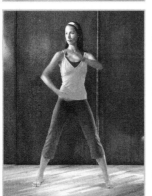

⊙ TWIST AND REACH

Step feet wide, arms wide and round (like you're holding a beach ball, right hand on top, left hand below). Shift weight to left, bending left knee slightly as you twist torso to right, raising left hand, palm up across body toward ceiling and lowering right, palm down, toward floor behind you, arms in a diagonal line.

Glide hands back to start position, opposite hand on top.

Then shift right and twist to left, switching arms. Alternate sides for 6 to 9 reps on each.

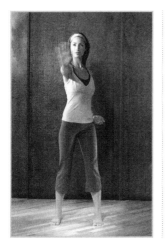

⊙ PUSH AND PULL

With feet hip-width apart, bend elbows so arms are at sides, palms facing each other. Simultaneously push right arm forward, palm facing away from you (like stopping traffic) and pull left hand back by hip, elbow behind you and palm facing up. Now pull right hand back and push left hand forward. Slowly continue to alternate hands for 6 to 9 reps with each arm. End by gently shaking out arms and legs (like doing the Hokey Pokey), then come to stillness, resting right hand on top of left, just below navel. Hold this position as long as you like.

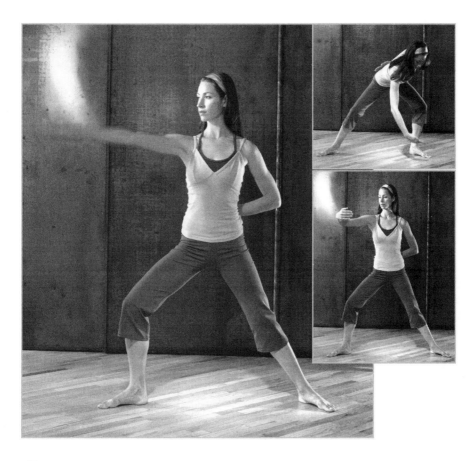

⌃ SCOOPING THE EARTH

Beginning with feet wide apart and toes turned out, rest back of left hand on lower back and extend right arm to side, parallel to floor, palm facing downward. Bend right knee into a lunge.

Hinge forward from hips, reaching right hand toward floor. Slowly shift weight to center (both legs equally bent in a plié squat), then to left side (lunging with left leg), scooping right arm across floor.

Inhaling, with left knee still bent, lift upper body, right arm stretched across body to left side, then slowly pull hand across front of body, exhaling and lunging to right. Eyes focus on right hand throughout. Do 6 to 9 times without stopping. Switch sides and repeat.

CHAPTER 21

MEND
Your Mood

How we think and what we do can intensify, even prolong, the best moments in life. Here's how to tune in to the small stuff and reap huge rewards!

Rose Theis is the consummate amateur athlete. Some might call her a machine. At age 46, she is an Ironman triathlete, an experienced marathoner, and a year-round bicyclist, which is a notable feat for a resident of Madison, Wisconsin, where the winters are no joke.

In the summer, Rose thinks nothing of awakening before dawn for a swim in the cool waters of Madison's Lake Monona. She isn't stopped by minor pains or by driving rains. But a school of muskies jumping upstream to spawn . . . a clump of magnolias spreading their flowering arms . . . a hot-pink sunrise looming over a glassy lake—those are pleasures worth stopping for.

Rose understands implicitly what Loyola University Chicago social psychologist Fred B. Bryant, PhD, wishes he could impart to all of us: Finding joy means opening yourself up to it. The value of taking time to appreciate positive experiences seems obvious—trite, even. Yet it's a skill that few people have mastered. The reason is simple: We're busy, and we have a lot on our minds. There'll always be other sunrises, we say to ourselves, but if we don't hit the shower soon, we'll never beat the traffic to work. Under the weight of our daily responsibilities and worries, we reflexively tune out the fleeting, spontaneous events that can happen at any time and that, if we let them, could bring us deeper joy and greater health.

For more than 20 years, Dr. Bryant has worked to understand what he terms mindful savoring: the things we think and do to intensify or prolong positive feelings.

"We all know people who are like this," Dr. Bryant says. "They're the life of the party, and they're the first people you want to turn to when something good happens. What is their gift?" Across the different cultures that Dr. Bryant has studied, women tend to possess this skill more often than do men.

Mindful savoring doesn't only enhance our feeling of well-being, Dr. Bryant notes. It might also improve health. A substantial body of related research indicates that people with a sunnier outlook about growing older recover more quickly from illness and live longer—$7\frac{1}{2}$ years on average, according to a large Yale University study—than people who have bleaker views. People who scored

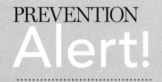

PREVENTION Alert!

SPREAD THE HAPPINESS VIRUS

Jotting down just five things you're grateful for every day can lead to a healthier mental state, research shows—and a Web site called ButterBeeHappy.com makes this route to joy easier than ever. Tools on the site include the Honeycomb, which looks for postings from people whose happy thoughts are similar to yours (users say it reinforces their own good feelings); a call-in "Happiness Hotline," where you can record an upbeat message for an online podcast; and a blog with the latest news in happiness research. Use of the site is free.

highest on a test Dr. Bryant designed that measures savoring ability also reported fewer illnesses.

Needless to say, it's easiest to appreciate the good when fortune leans in our favor. But when we're ill or anxious or beset by tragedy, savoring positive events is all the more important. Happiness, Dr. Bryant says, broadens our perspective and helps us recognize ways to cope with adversity.

"Bad things will come. We can't avoid them," he says. As many a poet has written, joy is fleeting, and elusive. "But if you know how, you can go hunting for joy, and you can make it last."

Here are 10 surefire strategies that Dr. Bryant says everyone can use to discover pleasure and satisfaction in everyday moments.

Share positive feelings. Let your children know how great it feels to spend time with them. Tell your spouse about the compliment your boss paid you. E-mail your best friend to tell her how fondly you remember the camping trip you took last year, and include a silly picture.

Sharing happy memories and experiences with others—or even simply anticipating doing so—is one of the most powerful and effective ways to prolong and magnify joy, Dr. Bryant's research shows. "It helps sustain emotions that would otherwise fade," he says. Affirming connections with others, he adds, is "the glue that holds people together."

Build memories. Take mental photographs of memorable moments that you can draw on later. Recall vivid, specific events, and pinpoint what brought you joy. Do you love your red wool scarf because it's stylish and warm, or because its smell reminds you of your childhood romps in the snow?

Just be careful not to overanalyze and lose the wonder of the moment. What you want, says University of Virginia social psychologist Timothy D. Wilson, PhD, is to dissect your experiences just enough to appreciate how they've helped form you and then get back to simply living them. Interjecting mystery into happy moments—reflecting on what's surprising or hard to understand about them, for example—can strengthen their power.

"If you analyze special times in a way that makes them seem ordinary or predictable, then you don't necessarily get as much benefit," Dr. Wilson says.

Congratulate yourself. Take pride in a hard-won accomplishment. If you spent a year sweating at the gym to reach a fitness goal, bask in your success—and share it with others such as family and friends. Self-congratulation doesn't come easily to everyone.

"A lot of people have trouble basking in an accomplishment because they feel that they shouldn't toot their own horns or rest on their laurels," Dr. Bryant says. It's a fine line between joyous self-congratulation and shameless self-promotion, but don't worry: You'll know if you're crossing it.

Fine-tune your senses. Close your eyes while you roll a square of dark chocolate over your tongue or fill your lungs with salty sea air or eavesdrop on your grandchildren's play and laughter. Shutting out some sensory stimuli while concentrating on others can heighten your enjoyment of positive experiences—particularly those that are short-lived.

Compare downward. Comparing upward makes us feel deprived, but comparing downward can heighten enjoyment. Think about how things could be worse—or how things used to be worse. Just keep it light; you don't have to relive your cancer diagnosis or revel in a neighbor's misfortune. Simply take note: Is today sunnier than promised? Are you fitter than you were a year ago?

Get absorbed. Some joyful moments seem to call for conscious reflection and dissection. At other times, we savor best when we simply immerse ourselves in the present moment, without deliberate analysis or judgment. Listen to your favorite music with headphones in a dark room. Lose yourself in a novel. Set aside enough time on the weekend for your favorite hobby so you can attain a level of absorption known as the "flow" state.

Fake it till you make it. Putting on a happy face—even if you don't feel like it—actually induces greater happiness, says Dr. Bryant. So be exuberant. Don't just eat the best peach of the season—luxuriate in every lip-smacking mouthful. Laugh aloud at the movies. Smile at yourself in the mirror. After all, he says, "a surefire way to kill joy is to suppress it."

Seize the moment. Some positive events come and go quickly—a surprise toast to your accomplishments at work, your daughter's sweet 16 party. It seems obvious that the more quickly a positive experience evaporates, the more difficult it is to savor. Yet paradoxically, Dr. Bryant has found, reminding ourselves that time is fleeting and joy transitory prompts us to seize positive moments while they last.

Avoid killjoy thinking. The world has enough pessimists. Short-circuit negative thoughts that can dampen enjoyment, such as self-recriminations or worries about others' perceptions. When you find yourself awash in happiness, give it space to grow. Don't ruminate about why you don't deserve this good thing, what could go wrong, how things could be better. Consciously make the decision to embrace joy.

Say thank you. Cultivate an "attitude of gratitude," Dr. Bryant says. Pinpoint what you're happy about—a party invitation, a patch of shade—and acknowledge its source. It's not always necessary to outwardly express gratitude, Dr. Bryant notes, but saying "thank you" to a friend, a stranger, or the universe deepens our happiness by making us more aware of it.

CHAPTER 22

STRENGTHEN YOUR
Relationships

Prevention's Head Coach columnist, Thomas Crook, PhD, tells how to increase levels of bonding hormones, reduce stress, and nurture every relationship—and how to cope with grief when needed

BOOST YOUR OXYTOCIN

Earlier this year, my wife and I went on a 5-day cruise to Mexico with our children, their spouses, and our young grandkids. Observing my own close-knit clan, I began ruminating on how readily old family members forge deep bonds with new additions, such as grandchildren and daughters-in-law. As a neuroscientist, I wondered: What mechanism in the brain is responsible for forging these connections among not just kin but also friends, neighbors—even strangers?

I had a hunch the answer involved oxytocin, which is a brain hormone you may already know a little about, and I was right. Oxytocin induces uterine contractions during childbirth, spurs the release (or letdown) of milk in the nursing mother, and is responsible, at first touch, for her feelings of instant attachment to the newborn. But its benefits go way beyond mother-infant bonding: Oxytocin plays a big role in brokering all of our relationships (men have it, too), strengthening marriages, promoting enduring friendships, even engendering trust among strangers. Many of the health benefits we associate with strong social connections start with this brain chemical. It decreases corticosterone and other stress hormones and helps lower blood pressure. That's reason enough for you to learn how to take maximum advantage of it.

Oxytocin's nickname—"the love hormone"—is well earned: As with a mom and her baby, it's released in the brain in response to hugs, kisses, and caresses, as well as simple touching. It's the main driver of a hormonal feedback loop that accounts for much of marriage's proven health benefit. A hug prompts the release of oxytocin, leading to feelings of closeness, sexual intimacy, and the release of more oxytocin. In fact, orgasm produces a spike in the hormone to more than two times the normal level, accounting for the calming postcoital afterglow and greater bonding.

Oxytocin can even induce warmth between strangers. Paul Zak, PhD, of Claremont Graduate University, and colleagues found that study participants given the hormone (through a nasal spray) were more generous toward strangers and trusted them much more than those who did not receive oxytocin.

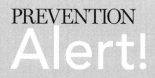

PREVENTION Alert!

PATCH UP YOUR LIBIDO

If your sex drive has cooled down—because of hormone abnormalities or surgery—a testosterone patch may help rekindle your fire. Over half of the 64 women who tried it in a University Hospitals of Cleveland study reported a big boost—nearly twice those with a placebo patch—resulting in four or five additional "satisfying" sexual episodes per month. Keep in mind: The patches are currently approved only for men, though about 20 percent are prescribed for women off-label.

The effects of this natural love potion are amplified by estrogen. That's one reason women tend to be more physically demonstrative than men (particularly during the high-estrogen days of the month when they're ovulating) and are generally more affected by touch. As estrogen declines during and after menopause, you'll want to take steps to ensure you continue to benefit from this life-enhancing hormone.

Here are some ways to do just that.

Surround yourself with positive people and avoid negative, hostile individuals.

Get physical, even if you're not in the mood. A few hugs and kisses will stimulate the release of oxytocin, which will get you there.

Muse about your romantic partner when apart. A University of North Carolina at Chapel Hill study showed that when women in good marriages were asked to think about their husbands, their oxytocin levels rose quickly.

Walk hand in hand, or arm in arm, with your spouse, children, and friends.

Adopt a pet: The love you feel for a dog or cat—or even a cute puppy you meet in the park—spurs the release of oxytocin.

RECOVER FROM GRIEF

Recently, my 58-year-old younger brother, a fit-and-sturdy Marine combat veteran, was diagnosed with lung cancer and died. Two weeks later, after an almost entirely disease-free life, I had to undergo eye surgery for cataracts.

THE PERCENTAGE OF DOCS WHO'D SWITCH FEMALE TESTOSTERONE-PATCH PATIENTS TO ONE APPROVED FOR WOMEN, ACCORDING TO *DATAMONITOR*, JUNE 2007

Since then, I've been thinking a lot about the inevitable setbacks we all encounter and how our brains deal with them.

Researchers completed an intriguing study recently that illustrates just how profound and widespread the effect of negative personal events can be. Three finance professors from major business schools tracked the performance of 75,000 Danish companies in the 2 years before and after the CEO had experienced a family death. Financial performance declined 20 percent after the loss of a child, 15 percent after the death of a spouse, and almost 10 percent after the demise of any other family member.

Indeed, when brain imaging studies are done on people who are grieving, increased activity is seen along a broad network of neurons. These link areas associated not only with mood but also with memory, perception, conceptualization, and even the regulation of the heart, the digestive system, and other organs. This shows the pervasive impact loss or even disappointment can have. And the more we dwell on negative thoughts, the more developed these neural pathways become. The result can be chronic preoccupation, sadness, or even depression.

So how can we learn to deal with loss, disappointment, and everyday setbacks more constructively? Keep in mind the following coping strategies, which are working for me.

Be on the alert for "intruders." As soon as you recognize an intrusive negative thought, visualize a stop sign. Even go so far as to say "Stop!" if it helps. Or try wearing a rubber band around your wrist and snap yourself out of it.

Schedule your sad memories. Just as you don't immediately indulge every pang of hunger, put off sad remembrances for a time when you don't need to be productive or engaged (say, during your lunch hour). Never examine such thoughts before bed, however. This is an invitation for negativity and blame to gather strength. Prior to sleep, electrical activity diminishes in brain regions associated with analytical reasoning, and we become less objective.

Don't tolerate self-accusing or superstitious thoughts. Examples of these would be "If only I had been . . . " or "Bad things happen in threes." Such thinking has no logical basis or benefit.

View setbacks as opportunities. Effectively dealing with difficulties that don't incapacitate you will make you stronger.

Don't be a "grieving widow" if you don't feel like one. Doing so will only make you feel guilty as you deal successfully with the loss.

Finally, keep in mind that during these emotionally vulnerable times, we all create illusions. We focus almost exclusively on how wonderful those who've disappeared from our lives made us feel, and we convince ourselves that no one could ever affect us like that again. I miss my brother, no doubt about it. I know that I can't avoid illness and death in my life, but I can choose how to deal with them. I'm lucky to have known my brother for 58 years, but I'm not going to dwell on the thought that our time together could have been longer.

PUTTING THE QUALITY IN TIME

After 3 months alone with his daughter, writer Joe Kita learned togetherness happens when you least expect it.

Quality time: It's the holy grail of modern parenthood. Mothers and fathers all over agree that it's essential for shaping a child's character, strengthening those family bonds, and insuring against multiple facial piercings. But beyond such generalities, there's a surprising lack of consensus about its nuances. Is there a difference between spending quality time and just spending time? And as children become young adults, does the chance for quality time start to run out?

I don't have a doctorate in any of this, but I did recently conduct some intensive research. Through a massive stroke of good fortune, I landed a teaching job on a cruise ship that visited 45 countries in 109 days—and I took my 18-year-old daughter, Claire, along as my guest. We threw snowballs in Antarctica. We learned to surf in the Indian Ocean, and we touched the pyramids, the Wailing Wall, and Jesus' tomb. We comforted each other after a robbery in Cape Town, and we damn near got arrested in Athens one muggy afternoon.

Indeed, I spent more quality time with my teenager than most parents ever will. What I learned is that it's still possible to connect with your kids years after the bedtime stories have been tucked in. And you don't even have to book a world cruise to do so. Here are a few lessons from our 3 months of together time.

BE THE BOSS. Teenagers are indecisive. They spend their days in the land of I Don't Know. My daughter initially turned up her nose at the offer of an around-the-world trip. She said she'd never be able to finish high school early (she did) and that she'd miss her friends too much (she didn't). So I forced her to go. Well, maybe *forced* is too strong a word. I told her it was a once-in-a-lifetime opportunity to meet cute Brazilian guys and generally lie around doing nothing.

TO GET QUALITY, GO FOR QUANTITY. The mere fact that I was with my daughter for such a long stretch guaranteed we'd have some special moments. This may be the shotgun approach to parenting, but it's simple and effective. The mistake parents often make is not spending enough overall time with their kids, then trying to make what little time they do share memorable. That's much harder to pull off. Relax. Just hang out.

DO MORE, TALK LESS. Quality time, to a teenager, is never going to involve a mellow evening of conversation in the parlor. They prefer *doing* to *being*. In Walvis Bay, Namibia, along the coast of Africa, we rented sea kayaks. We unexpectedly paddled into a large group of seals, who played with our sleek shells as if we were long-lost members of the herd. My daughter and I never said a word to each other while it was happening, but this is one of our fondest memories. Doing things together, even if you are doing them separately, is powerful glue.

TREAT THEM LIKE ADULTS. Kids want nothing more than to grow up, so they'll relish any moment their maturity is recognized. Claire and I went to dinner one night on the ship—just us, no usual table of eight. I wore a tuxedo, and she was bejeweled and beautiful. We talked about the trip and about life. (She admitted being apprehensive about college but said she was looking forward to the parties.) She opened up, and I realized the importance of treating my baby like a young lady.

BUT WALK IN THEIR FLIP-FLOPS. I didn't want to be in Rio de Janeiro's famed Sambódromo at 3 AM during Carnival surrounded by drunken Brazilians while being pummeled by a sound system that could be heard in Argentina. But Claire did. When a teenager peeks out from the land of I Don't Know and invites you in, never think you're too old or tired. Instead, seize the moment (and down a Red Bull if you have to).

LET GO A LITTLE. The cruise was scheduled to conclude just in time for Claire's prom, so she wanted to buy a gown in some exotic town—Buenos Aires, it turns out. I hadn't shopped for dresses with my daughter since she was 6, so I let the boutique owner take over. When Claire emerged from the dressing room, she was sporting a backless blue satin gown with a plunging neckline. Although that dress didn't match the vision I had of my little girl, I bought it anyway. Letting your kids pursue their dreams makes you a part of them.

GIVE 'EM SOME SPACE. One day, my daughter and I were sunning on the deck. An older man tottered over, squinted down at us, and said: "You're such a lovely couple; I hope you enjoy your honeymoon." His eyesight probably didn't register the age difference, but my daughter gagged on her iced tea and from then on, sat two chairs down from mine. So yes, it is possible to spend too much quality time together. Fortunately, you can just do what we did and create a little quality space.

CHAPTER 23

Mind Over MALADY

Meditation has a profound effect on health, mood, even how you eat. Here are four new ways to tap into the new "mindfulness"—and reap its rewards today

Once the catchphrase of 1960s counterculture, "mindfulness" has finally graduated from the fringe to the mainstream. "Staying in the moment" is now the guiding principle of millions of devotees who faithfully practice mindfulness meditation to enrich their daily lives.

Just as impressively, mindfulness has also attracted another group of admirers: clinical researchers, whose latest investigations document its surprising and powerful physical and mental health benefits—achieved in as little as 5 minutes a day.

For example, mindfulness meditation—paying close attention to your thoughts, feelings, actions, and body sensations in an objective, nonattached way—is a proven pain reliever. Here's how it works: Pain has not only sensory dimensions (ouch!) but also emotional and cognitive ones—the turbulent thoughts and feelings ("This is killing me") that accompany discomfort.

"When you zero in on the pain with kind, nonjudgmental attention, you separate the emotional and cognitive elements from the sensory ones," explains Jon Kabat-Zinn, PhD, professor of medicine emeritus at the University of Massachusetts and the founder of mindfulness-based stress reduction (MBSR). "And because you're not identifying with all those turbulent thoughts, and you recognize that the sensations are just sensations—however unpleasant— for that moment, there can be significantly less suffering. When you focus attention in this way, it causes special areas of the brain to tamp down on the signals that are interpreted as pain."

Mindfulness works by interrupting learned behavior, which is one reason it also helps treat compulsive habits, such as binge eating. Because the practice enables you to observe your actions without judging them, it short-circuits the process that connects stress with eating, explains Ruth Q. Wolever, PhD, research director at Duke Integrative Medicine. Once the binge eater is emotionally separated from her usual response, she can see that there are healthier ways to deal with these urges.

Researchers have also learned that brief mindfulness meditation sessions improve memory and attention, ease anxiety—even deepen personal relationships. You can learn more about mindfulness meditation and its many benefits at prevention.com/calm. Here are four proven health boosts you, too, can receive by simply learning how to "stay in the moment."

GAIN CONTROL OVER EMOTIONAL EATING

A recent NIH-funded study tracked the eating patterns of 140 binge eaters (people who eat excessively and rapidly while feeling a loss of control, but don't purge). Researchers found that those using mindfulness-based interventions reduced their bingeing from about four times to once per week. The mindfulness group also reported feeling more in control around food than study participants who received only support and education.

Try this technique: Raisin Meditation (5 minutes): This exercise is designed to interrupt the emotional connection you may have with food. Hold one raisin (or other favorite snack) and look it over as if you've never seen one before. Notice how the fruit feels between your fingers, and take in its colors and ridges. Inhale its scent. Simply notice any thoughts you may have (for instance, like or dislike) without trying to push them away. Finally, bring the raisin to your lips, observing the movement of your hand and arm, and notice how you salivate in anticipation of eating the morsel. Chew slowly, taking in the taste. Observe the impulse to swallow as it wells up, then make the conscious decision that you will now do so.

BOOST YOUR SPIRITS—AND IMMUNITY

Mindfulness meditation eases anxiety by 44 percent and reduces symptoms of depression by 34 percent while simultaneously jacking up immunity. In a study of stressed biotech employees, Richard Davidson, PhD, and his colleagues at the University of Wisconsin, along with Dr. Kabat-Zinn, found that those who completed an 8-week MBSR program had a significantly higher level of activity in the left prefrontal cortex (the brain region associated with a happy, calm state) than colleagues who received no training. At the end of the program, both groups were given flu vaccines, followed by blood tests. Results: The meditators produced significantly more antibodies than the nonmeditators.

Try this technique: Mindful Walking (10 minutes): Pick a quiet place, such as your bedroom or living room, where you can walk slowly back and forth or in circles. Looking straight ahead, focus on one aspect of walking. For example, home in on your feet: Notice how one foot makes contact with the ground; your weight shifts; and the other foot lifts, moves forward, and finally makes contact. Continue to direct your attention toward your feet, and whenever your mind wanders, gently bring it back.

EASE PAIN

Mindfulness meditation helps older adults better cope with chronic pain in the lower back, according to a University of Pittsburgh study. Adults over age 65 with almost daily lower-back pain who participated in an 8-week mindfulness meditation program, in which they reported meditating an average of 4 days a week, improved their physical function (carrying groceries, for exam-

---

TRAIN YOURSELF TO BE MINDFUL

Try these simple techniques to be more in the moment.
- Every hour, stop whatever you're doing and focus on your breathing for 60 seconds.
- Savor each bite of your food during meals, and eliminate distractions, such as TV.
- During a strength-training exercise, close your eyes for 1 set of repetitions and concentrate on the movement of your body.

ple). Anecdotally, two patients in the study stopped using their walking canes; and at a 3-month follow-up, a third of the subjects reported taking fewer pain and/or sleep meds.

Try this technique: Body Scan (10 to 20 minutes): Lie comfortably on your back, side, or stomach with your eyes closed. Beginning with the toes of your left foot, focus on any sensations (tingling, warmth) you feel there. Now imagine your breath traveling down to your toes, then back up and out through your nose. Slowly move up your left leg, focusing on the sensations you encounter and directing your breath to your ankle, shin, knee, and thigh. Repeat the sequence with your right leg, then move through your lower back, abdomen, upper back, chest, shoulders, and both arms. Next move to your neck, throat, face, the back of your head, and—finally—the top of your head. You should also take notice when you don't feel any sensations at all.

STRENGTHEN RELATIONSHIPS

When you focus on new details in everyday activities and encounters, you're much more engaged, are viewed as more genuine, and, consequently, are more attractive to others. In a study by Ellen Langer, PhD, a Harvard psychologist and author of *The Power of Mindful Learning*, participants were asked to sell magazines either mindfully or mindlessly. Everyone memorized a sales pitch so they could recite it by rote. One group was asked to repeat the pitch verbatim with each new customer (i.e., mindlessly); the other group was told to change the script in subtle ways, such as pausing in different places (i.e., mindfully), so that only they knew how it differed each time. When the customers were asked their opinions of the salespeople, they judged the script changers (the mindful group) as more charismatic, says Dr. Langer.

A recent study from the University of North Carolina-Chapel Hill found that mindfulness techniques improve personal relationships as well. Couples who completed separate 8-week courses in traditional mindfulness-based techniques felt significantly more satisfied with their relationships than before; they also reported less stress within the relationship. These results were still in effect 3 months later.

Try this technique: Say Hello—Mindfully (10 minutes): The next time you get together with good friends, make every effort to notice new details about them (what they're wearing, the color of their eyes) and observe their physical reaction to you—and yours to them. Do you feel yourself retreating or opening toward the others? Do you sense they're defensive, or eager to foster greater intimacy? Later, take a few moments to review what you've learned and how that new info has altered your perceptions of your friends.

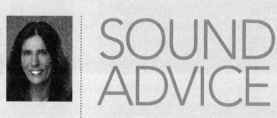

SOUND ADVICE

TOP THREE WAYS TO GET OUT OF A FUNK

What should you do when your hue is too blue? We asked Tieraona Low Dog, MD, director of education of the Program in Integrative Medicine at the University of Arizona, one of *Prevention*'s complementary and alternative medicine advisors. She suggests the following tricks; combine as many of them as you can.

1. TEND AND BEFRIEND. Often when people feel blue or down, they want to curl up in a ball on the couch and watch TV, says Dr. Low Dog. But especially for women, that's the worst thing you can do. While men have a fight-or-flight response to stress, women are programmed to reach out, socialize, and connect with other people during times of stress. So if you're feeling sad, don't isolate yourself. Instead, call a friend or make plans to meet for tea or a movie.

2. GO FOR A WALK. It's best if you can walk outside because then you have the benefit of exercise and sunlight, says Dr. Low Dog. Exercise has been shown to be as effective as antidepressants for mood. But if it's too cold or too hot to go outside, go walk at a mall. This will get you out of the house and give you a safe, comfortable place to walk. Then, after a few laps, get a Jamba Juice and do some people watching.

3. DO SOME RELAXATION PRACTICE. Just breathe, says Dr. Low Dog. If you don't know of a particular relaxation practice that works for you, it's a good time to find one. You can buy CDs on basic breathing such as Amy Weintraub's *Breathe to Beat the Blues*. You can use breath to help you to find your center. Better yet, listen to a CD while taking a bath. Best of all, listen to the CD while taking a bath with some citrus essential oil in it. It's energizing yet also calming, and it'll lift you up. It's like having your own spa.

Part6

BEAUTY
BREAKTHROUGHS

CHAPTER 24

LOOK YOUNGER ON A BUDGET

When economic times turn tough, it might seem that beauty indulgences should be the first things to go. But just because your budget calls for some belt tightening, that's no reason not to look better than ever. The trick is to bolster your beauty routine by making no- or low-cost moves that deliver maximum impact. From hiding dark circles to boosting hair's shine, here are experts' top tips for trimming costs—and a few years, to boot!

PUMP UP HAIR'S VOLUME

Switch to mousse. It costs the same as other styling products, but because it contains resins that lightly coat strands to add thickness and lift hair at the root, mousse delivers far more oomph, says Renee Cohen, senior stylist at Serge Normant at the John Frieda Salon in New York City.

Dry hair upside down. To build volume when you blow-dry, work a palm full of mousse from your roots through to the ends, then flip your head over and dry your hair away from the scalp. "Hair should be barely damp before you flip it back up and style it," she says.

Brush in fullness. Using a round brush to style hair builds in more volume. Pick a medium-size brush (for longer hair) or small (for shorter)—the full circle of bristles will give roots a lift as you blow-dry, brushing in the opposite direction the hair is going to lay. Hook the brush under a 2-inch section of hair at the root, and lift as you roll it through to the ends—all the while following the brush with the dryer. Keep the nozzle above your brush and pointed down to increase shine.

RESTORE LOCKS' LUSTER

Give yourself a weekly hot-oil treatment. Save a bundle by substituting jojoba oil (in natural food stores for about $10) for pricier hair-repair products.

"Jojoba has a fine molecular structure that allows it to enter and fill the hair shaft, making it a perfect choice for conditioning," says Paul Labrecque, owner of the New York City-based Paul Labrecque Salon. Spread the oil liberally through dry hair, put on a plastic shower cap, then cover with a hot towel for 30 minutes. Wash it out thoroughly, then rinse with cold water to seal the cuticle and trap added moisture. "When the hair shaft is infused with oil, the cuticle lies flatter, so your hair looks smoother and shinier," he explains.

Keep a cool head. Heat opens hair's protective outer layer, damaging strands and creating frizz. "Frequently cooling the hair while styling helps keep your cuticle flat," says Labrecque. If your dryer has a cool-shot button, use it to deliver a blast of cold air after drying each individual section. (This

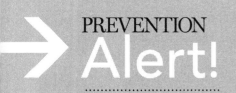

PREVENTION
Alert!

LOW-CAL WRINKLE REDUCER
Not only are clementines portable and easy to peel, but two contain only 70 calories and a whopping 96 percent of your daily need for wrinkle-reducing vitamin C.

also helps lock in your new style.) If it doesn't, he suggests holding your style in place with your brush for about 30 seconds to let hair cool off.

SOOTHE SKIN

Get milk. Soak a clean washcloth in cold milk and place it over your face for 10 minutes.

"Milk contains proteins, fat, amino acids, and vitamin A—all of which reduce redness and calm irritated skin," says David Bank, MD, a dermatologist in Mount Kisco, New York. Bonus: The lactic acid in milk exfoliates, so skin looks soft and glowing.

Banish brown spots. Camouflage with care. First, dab concealer that's one or two shades lighter than your foundation onto the spot. Use a concealer brush. It'll give more precise coverage than your finger. Follow with a dot of foundation that exactly matches your skin tone.

"The concealer lightens the spot, and the foundation helps blend it seamlessly," says New York City–based makeup artist Jessica Liebeskind.

Replace your makeup wisely. "Switching from powder formulas to creamier ones gives your skin a soft reflective sheen," says Kimara Ahnert, a makeup artist in New York City. Cheeks tend to be drier than your T-zone, so as soon as you use up your powder blush, buy a light liquid or cream formula that imparts a youthful glow instead of leaving skin dull and matte.

PLUMP THIN LIPS

Think pink. "Dark or bright colors call attention to the size of your lips, emphasizing thinness and fine lines around your mouth," says Liebeskind. Instead, choose a lipstick that mimics the color that your lips were when you were younger.

Define your lips. After applying your lipstick, line just at the outer edge of the natural border of your mouth with a pencil in a shade that exactly matches your lipstick. Don't try to draw on a bigger pout. It'll only look fake.

BRIGHTEN YOUR SMILE

Mix your own whitener. Brushing with a paste made of baking soda and water a few times a month removes superficial staining and whitens teeth by a shade or two. "The graininess neutralizes stains and polishes teeth but isn't abrasive enough to wear down your enamel," says Jennifer Jablow, DDS, a cosmetic dentist in New York City.

Keep teeth whiter, longer. To sidestep stains when drinking red wine, chase your vino with a handful of crunchy raw vegetables. "They have a brushing action that can rub away newly setting stains," says Jablow.

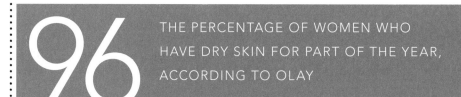

96 THE PERCENTAGE OF WOMEN WHO HAVE DRY SKIN FOR PART OF THE YEAR, ACCORDING TO OLAY

WARD OFF WRINKLES IN A FLASH

A new British Skin Foundation study finds that 50 percent of women don't wash their faces at night, a habit that can make you look older.

"Leaving dirt, excess oil, and makeup on overnight can enlarge pores and further irritate dry skin," says Robin Ashinoff, MD, a dermatologist at Hackensack University Medical Center in New Jersey.

To suds away signs of aging, gently rub facial cleanser onto damp skin for 2 minutes and rinse 10 times with lukewarm water.

Choose the right lipstick shade. "Colors with blue undertones make teeth appear brighter," explains Liebeskind. To figure out which of your lipsticks fit the bill, she recommends lining up three or four shades. In comparison to each other, it will be more obvious which are blue-based and which have yellow or gold undertones that bring out the yellow in teeth.

MINIMIZE UNDER-EYE CIRCLES

Be generous with your concealer. "The biggest mistake women make is using too little concealer," says Liebeskind. Start by putting on eye cream. Concealer can settle into fine lines of all skin types, especially drier complexions. Then apply a generous layer of concealer from the inner corner of the eye around to the outer corner with a concealer brush. Pat and press the product into the skin to blend. If there's still any darkness visible, apply a second layer of concealer. Set the concealer with a dusting of face powder that matches your foundation.

Caffeinate your eyes. Tea bags can perk up tired-looking eyes. "The caffeine helps shrink the underlying dark blood vessels and forces out some of the liquid that creates puffiness," explains Ava Shamban, MD, assistant clinical professor of dermatology at UCLA. Soak tea bags in hot water for a minute before plunging them into ice water for a few seconds. Lie down and apply them directly to your eyes for 15 minutes.

SMOOTH WRINKLES

Keep makeup outside the lines. To be sure there's no excess makeup to settle into—and emphasize—the fine lines around your eyes and mouth, Ahnert suggests using a dry makeup sponge to gently smooth and blend makeup after applying it. Don't wipe, though, or you'll rub it off.

GIVE EYES A LIFT

Curl lashes correctly. When lashes are clean and dry (wet ones won't hold a curl), position the curler at the root of lashes and give three firm, gentle pumps. Release and repeat. "Holding it steady doesn't create a natural-looking, fluid curl," says Liebeskind.

Create a long-lasting curl. Heat your curler with your blow-dryer for 15 seconds first. "The warmth holds the bend better," says NYC–based makeup artist Mally Roncal.

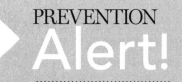

PREVENTION
Alert!

SURPRISE DRY SKIN CULPRIT

Here's a good reason to step up your housecleaning: Dust mites can increase skin sensitivity, finds a new study in the *Journal of Investigative Dermatology.*

South Korean researchers say exposure to the microscopic bugs prolongs inflammation and irritation, making it harder for people who suffer from conditions such as eczema to heal. Carpets and sheets harbor the most dust mites, so vacuum floors and wash your bedding weekly in 130°F water.

YOUR GLOWING SKIN PLAN

Daily

WORK OUT. Exercise 3 or 4 days a week to decrease tension, boost circulation, and keep inflammation in check.

"Even a long walk can pump out positive endorphins," says Richard Fried, MD, PhD, a dermatologist and psychologist in Yardley, Pennsylvania.

CATCH ENOUGH ZZZS. Sleeping less than 7 to 8 hours a night not only monkeys with your mood, but causes the body to release cortisol, increasing dryness and inflammation, says Amy Wechsler, MD, a dermatologist and psychiatrist in New York City and author of *The Mind-Beauty Connection*.

Weekly

KEEP A SKIN DIARY. "Write down what's going on in your life when your skin acts up and when it gets better," Dr. Wechsler says. That helps you zero in on the emotional issue that's triggering your skin problem.

When Desperate

SEE A SKIN SHRINK. Consider seeing a dermatologist who's also board certified in psychiatry or psychology, known as psychodermatologists. Besides prescribing antibiotics for acne and retinoids for wrinkles, they will recommend alternative techniques such as acupuncture and massage.

CHAPTER 25

Keep Stress Off
YOUR FACE

New research shows that worrying and a high-pressure lifestyle can damage your dermis. Here are new strategies to restore your smooth, even glow, plus nature's fixes for flawless skin

Stress is not for the faint of heart—nor thin of skin. You know at some gut level (like when you catch the reflection of your furrowed brow in a window) that stress doesn't help your appearance. Now science is detailing the myriad ways the stress hormone cortisol literally gets under your skin, leading to dryness and other signs of aging (including, yes, those lovely worry lines).

But what science reveals it also heals. Once you identify how your inner turmoil shows itself, you can use targeted home and pro therapies to counter its not-so-pretty effects. With our strategies, your skin will look calm, cool, and collected—and so will you.

STRESS SYMPTOM: DRYNESS

"Chronic stress increases the hormone cortisol, which damages skin's ability to hold on to water," says Peter Elias, MD, a professor of dermatology at the University of California, San Francisco. The resulting moisture loss also diminishes luminosity, explains David Goldberg, MD, a clinical professor of dermatology and director of laser research at Mount Sinai School of Medicine.

Correct It

Look for hypoallergenic, fragrance-free products. "Their lower pH prevents further dryness and inflammation," says Dr. Goldberg. Wash your face with lukewarm water; hot temperatures strip skin's oils. Slathering on your face cream while skin is slightly damp traps moisture.

STRESS SYMPTOM: FINE LINES

Cortisol triggers an elevation in blood sugar, which—via a process called glycation—damages collagen and elastin, the protein fibers that plump skin and keep it smooth. Constant muscle tension also leads to permanent wrinkling.

Correct It

OTC creams made with retinol and antioxidants encourage collagen production to firm skin. An Rx retinoid like Renova offers significantly better results. For an instant fix, you can soften lines by relaxing muscles with Botox (costs around $400 per treated area and lasts up to 4 months) or filling them in with injectables such as Evolence or Restylane ($600 and up, with results lasting 6 months).

STRESS SYMPTOM: REDNESS

The increased bloodflow that occurs when you're under duress may cause capillaries to expand. Stress also triggers flushing known as rosacea, according to the National Rosacea Society. And because stress weakens your immune system, flare-ups may last longer.

Correct It

When used daily, topical creams made with anti-inflammatories such as allantoin and licorice root extract can ease ruddiness. Rx treatment includes light and laser therapy that zap blood vessels: You'll need several sessions that each cost $300 and up. If you suffer from rosacea, you may need topical prescriptions to reduce inflammation.

MYSTERY SPOTS, EXPLAINED

If you're seeing dark patches above the lip, on the forehead, or along the temples, you may have melasma. A boost in estrogen from pregnancy, hormone therapy, or birth control pills is the most likely culprit. Melasma may clear once hormones stabilize, but treatment is usually needed.

The OTC potions that fade sun spots deliver modest improvement. A more potent Rx bleacher such as Tri-Luma (with 4% hydroquinone, a retinoid, and a skin-calming cortisone) often delivers complete clearing after 3 months.

For stubborn cases, a fractionated laser like Fraxel can erase discoloration after four to six sessions at $1,130 per visit. UV exposure exacerbates melasma, so protect skin daily with sunscreen.

STRESS SYMPTOM: ACNE

Stress increases the inflammation that leads to breakouts, says Gil Yosipo-vitch, MD, a clinical professor of dermatology at Wake Forest University.

Correct It

Use a lotion containing skin-sloughing salicylic acid or bacteria-busting ben-zoyl peroxide, plus a noncomedogenic moisturizer so skin won't get too dry. If your skin doesn't respond to treatment within a few weeks, see your doctor for more potent meds.

STRESS SYMPTOM: TIRED EYES

Anxiety causes a chain reaction, leading to sleepless nights, which in turn cause puffiness, says Amy Wechsler, MD, a dermatologist and psychiatrist in New York City and author of *The Mind-Beauty Connection*.

Correct It

Use cucumber slices as mini ice packs for the eyes; they constrict the blood and lymph vessels that bring fluid to the area. Sleep with your head slightly elevated to prevent fluid from pooling.

ANTI-AGING MAKEUP REMOVERS

A new generation of cleansing cloths does more than wash away the day: Infused with youth boosters such as glycerin, retinol, and vitamin C, these disposable towelettes hydrate, plump creases, and even help fade sun spots. For best results, rub in a gentle circular motion and follow with a light layer of moisturizer to seal in the beneficial ingredients.

Try: L'Oréal Paris Revitalift Radiant Smoothing Wet Cleansing Towelettes ($7), Bioré Refresh Daily Cleansing Cloths ($6), and Pond's Clean Sweep Wet Cleansing Towelettes in Age Defying ($6). All are available at drugstores.

90

NATURE'S FIXES FOR FLAWLESS SKIN

We're not surprised that the latest crop of skin rejuvenators comes straight from Mother Nature. Many of you prefer products that harness the anti-aging power of plants and believe they're better for your skin. Doctors say they're effective, too.

"Botanicals are the best sources for discovering new ingredients that protect and repair aging skin," says Zoe Draelos, MD, a clinical and research dermatologist in High Point, North Carolina. Vitamins, antioxidants, and emollients that spring from leaves, nuts, and fruits can soften wrinkles, fight sagging, and boost radiance. Here, we've unearthed five that deliver a major youth boost—just how nature intended.

Bearberry

A flowering shrub that flourishes throughout the United States, bearberry is quickly becoming a popular skin brightener. The leaves contain arbutin, which is a derivative of the skin lightener hydroquinone, which reduces the formation of pigment-producing melanin. Unfortunately, HQ can irritate skin. Bearberry is a milder—but effective—HQ alternative when combined with other botanically based pigment faders, says Sonia Badreshia-Bansal, MD, a dermatologist in San Francisco.

In one study published in the *Journal of Investigative Dermatology*, women with melasma who applied a cocktail that included bearberry extract once a day lightened the dark patches of skin by nearly 70 percent after 3 months—without any side effects. Those using prescription-strength HQ saw a 77 percent improvement, but a quarter of them reported reactions, such as itchy skin.

(continued on page 330)

SEE SPOTS RUN

When Lady Macbeth cries, "Out, damn'd spot!" the mark she berates is marring her conscience—not her complexion. Lucky her. A lifetime of sun exposure means that the spots on your face are probably as plain as day.

"This discoloration doesn't discriminate. It's a problem that all women over 40 eventually develop," says Susan Taylor, MD, director of the Skin of Color Center at St. Luke's-Roosevelt Hospital in New York City.

Even if skin is wrinkle free, the resulting spots can add years to your look, making others view you as unhealthy and up to 10 years older, according to recent research. Still, spots needn't drive you mad. Whether you want to treat them yourself or visit a pro, a range of remedies—from bleaching agents to high-tech lasers—will help you see speckled skin isn't a tragedy after all.

THE MOST IMPORTANT STEP TO PREVENTING SPOTS: Apply a broad-spectrum sunscreen with an SPF of at least 15 (30 is best) every day. This blocks the UV rays that speed up the production of melanin, the pigment that gives skin color. For extra protection, layer it over a cream or lotion that contains an antioxidant such as green tea, coffee berry, or vitamin C.

AT-HOME FIXES: OTC options may take months to show improvement, but they're budget friendly and the least irritating.

Step 1: Apply a product with 2 percent hydroquinone directly onto spots. The most potent skin lightener, HQ suppresses the enzyme needed for melanin production. Diligent nightly application can result in complete clearing of mild to moderate spots within 4 weeks, says Heather Woolery-Lloyd, MD, an assistant professor of dermatology at the University of Miami School of Medicine. One caveat: Even low doses of HQ can cause irritation. To lower the risk, start by applying every other evening and build up to nightly use.

Step 2: Once spots subside, switch to a cream with glucosamine or niacinamide (a B vitamin) to maintain results.

Consider Sepiwhite. This new nonirritating bleacher for mild mottling does double duty: It suppresses the production of melanin and its migration into skin cells, explains Jeffrey Dover, MD, a clinical associate professor of dermatology at Yale University. Studies show that Sepiwhite significantly increases luminosity and lightens spots in 2 months. For even faster clearing, use an exfoliator with retinol or glycolic acid to drive any bleacher deeper into skin.

IN-OFFICE SOLUTIONS: Although more costly, Rx remedies are faster, sometimes immediate, solutions.

Step 1: Use an Rx retinoid nightly to speed cell turnover and even skin tone.

Step 2: Pair your retinoid with an Rx 4% HQ cream. The combo can eliminate the most severe spots in as little as 4 to 6 weeks. Both ingredients are irritating, so use as advised. To avoid worsening discoloration, apply for no longer than 60 days in a row three times a year, says Dr. Taylor.

Consider microdermabrasion or chemical peels. They even out mottling by polishing skin's surface or dissolving dead cells. Plan on three to five treatments at about $200 a pop.

Consider light therapy. Intense pulsed light therapy (IPL) offers the fastest fix, zapping away both brown and red pigment, making it ideal for women who also have broken capillaries or ruddiness.

"The light superficially burns the spots and makes them a bit darker for a couple of days," says Dr. Woolery-Lloyd. "They peel off in less than a week, revealing fresh skin." Depending on the severity of your discoloration, you'll need three to six monthly treatments at about $250 a session. Expect slight stinging and redness that disappears within a few days.

Find it in: Exuviance Essential Skin Brightening Gel ($21.50; exuviance. com), Derma-doctor Immaculate Correction ($62; dermadoctor.com), June Jacobs Redness Diffusing Serum ($60; junejacobs.com), and Juice Beauty Soothing Serum ($36; juicebeauty.com).

Acai

It may be little, but this brightly colored Brazilian berry (pronounced ah-sigh-ee) packs a big anti-aging punch. Acai berries are rich in emollients such as essential fatty acids and phytosterols that help seal in moisture and strengthen the skin's surface so it's more resilient against outside irritation, says Howard Sobel, MD, a New York City dermatologist and founder of DDF Skincare.

Acai is a powerful protector against free radicals, too. The pulp contains a significant concentration of anthocyanins, the antioxidant pigments that give red and purple produce their deep hue. Hence the reason this superfruit boasts one of the highest ORAC scores, thought to measure a food's ability to combat premature aging—even when applied on skin.

"Acai reduces UV damage that eventually causes wrinkles, brown spots,

---

THREE BEAUTY PICKS WE TRUST

There are loads out there that promise to make you look younger. Here are some new picks with proven results.

FOR NAILS: Studies find that the B vitamin biotin in Sally Hansen Nail Essentials Daily Supplement ($13; drugstores) significantly fortifies fragile nails.

FOR SUN PROTECTION: Packed with pomegranate extract, Murad Pomphenol Sunguard Dietary Supplement ($36; murad.com) is a proven wrinkle fighter.

FOR REDUCING BRUISING: Research shows that the bromelain and arnica montana in J PAK System No. 1 ($20; jpaksystems.com) lessen post-Botox bruising and swelling to speed healing.

and sagging," says Dr. Sobel. That's proof that good things really do come in small packages.

Find it in: Pangea Organics Japanese Matcha Tea with Acai & Gogi Berry Facial Mask ($35; pangeaorganics.com), Ikove Organic Acai Chocolate Facial Exfoliate ($20; Whole Foods), DDF Mesojection Healthy Cell Serum ($84; beauty.com), and Tarte Double Dose Berry Boost & Gloss in Acai Boost ($21; sephora.com).

Red Tea

Tea brewed from the leaves of this South African shrub is rich in anti-inflammatories such as quercetin that help relieve itchiness and facial flushing.

"Red tea is ideal for reducing irritation associated with rosacea and eczema flare-ups," says Petko Detchev, PhD, senior chemist at Jason Natural Products. It soothes skin after a peel or microdermabrasion, too.

Red tea also shines at preventing the UV damage that causes fine lines and brown spots. Packed with antioxidants—including aspalathin, found only in red tea—it reduces free radical damage by as much as 90 percent, according to one study. Red tea decreased skin cancer tumors at least 60 percent, as well.

Find it in: Jason Red Elements Red Clay Masque ($13.60; jason-natural.com), Care by Stella McCartney Radiance & Youth Elixir ($64; nordstrom.com), and Dermalogica Daily Resurfacer ($66; ulta.com).

Argan Oil

Pressed from the nut of the Moroccan argan tree, the oil is touted as "liquid gold" for its ability to moisturize dry, lackluster skin. A high concentration of essential fatty acids and vitamin E, two key parts of skin's lubricating layer, explains the oil's power.

"These two components help the skin stay hydrated and prevent further moisture loss," says Ni'Kita Wilson, a cosmetic chemist in Fairfield, New Jersey.

The leaves of the tree are loaded with glycerin, a humectant that attracts water, plumping wrinkles, says Pat Peterson, executive director of research and development at Aveda. The leaf extract fends off wrinkle-causing free radicals as well, reducing collagen and elastin damage by 45 percent in one study.

Find it in: Liz Earle Naturally Active Skincare Superskin Concentrate ($34; us.lizearle.com), Kiehl's Superbly Restorative Dry Oil ($30; kiehls.com), Kaeline Argatherapie Argarôme Jour Day Serum ($38; xandrarenouvelle.com), and Aveda Green Science Line Minimizer ($85; aveda.com).

Durian

Dubbed the King of Fruit in Asia, durian may soon rule the world as a top skin rejuvenator. Don't let its spiky exterior scare you: The source of durian's beauty benefits is the creamy pulp, which contains hydrating oils, protective antioxidants, and natural sugars that strengthen cell membranes and prevent moisture from escaping, says Howard Murad, MD, an associate clinical professor of dermatology at UCLA.

So far, durian is only available in one line: Find it in Murad Intensive Wrinkle Reducer for Eyes ($90; murad.com).

For more age-defying potions to help you look younger naturally, check out prevention.com/organicbeauty.

Are you looking for the best products for your skin? Then you probably rely on label claims such as fragrance free and hypoallergenic to help you in your hunt. The hitch: Despite widespread use, there are no standard definitions for such terms, and no one regulates how they should be employed. Some companies abide by their own strict interpretations, while others aren't as careful. Still, you don't want to discount them.

"Labels can give you a good starting point for picking the right products," says John Bailey, PhD, executive vice president of science at the Cosmetic, Toiletry, and Fragrance Association. So learn precisely what the jargon on your tubes and jars means—and doesn't mean. If information is power, this guide will make you queen of the beauty aisle.

Dermatologist Tested

YOU THINK IT MEANS: A skin specialist found the product to be effective and also nonirritating.

THE REALITY: Testing can vary widely. "A dermatologist may have given the product to staffers to try or she may have conducted a legitimate, controlled trial," says Ranella Hirsch, MD, president-elect of the American Society of Cosmetic Dermatology & Aesthetic Surgery.

WHEN IT'S DONE RIGHT: A large-scale study on carefully selected, randomized volunteers will have been carried out. Such meaningful testing is the norm for big brands such as Olay, Neutrogena, L'Oréal, and Vichy, which tested its Nutrilogie 2 Intensive Nourishing Moisturizer Cream on 114 women in four countries. Other tip-offs that the derm-tested claim is valid: The package insert may elaborate on the role the doctor played in testing, says Jeannette Graf, MD, an assistant professor of dermatology at New York University Medical Center, or the company may promote its relationship with a particular dermatologist.

(continued)

Fragrance Free

YOU THINK IT MEANS: The product is unscented and won't irritate skin.

THE REALITY: Fragrance free usually means that no scents were added, and this does reduce the likelihood that women with sensitive skin will have a reaction. Don't be surprised, though, if a fragrance-free product has an aroma. What you smell is the natural odor of the ingredients used to formulate the product, such as lavender (for its antiseptic properties) and grapefruit seed (a natural preservative). Products labeled unscented, on the other hand, do contain low levels—less than 1 percent—of fragrance, called masking agents, to cover up the sometimes unpleasant natural odor of raw materials, explains Yohini Appa, PhD, executive director of scientific affairs at Neutrogena.

WHEN IT'S DONE RIGHT: Companies are aware that it's usually women prone to fragrance sensitivities who shop for these products, so those containing any form of fragrance will have undergone a battery of safety checks to ensure that they don't irritate or cause allergic reactions. One company that goes above and beyond this standard is Almay, which doesn't use fragrances or masking agents in either its skin care or makeup lines. Still, despite a product's label, it's always a good idea to check for ingredients you know from previous experience might upset your skin.

Hypoallergenic

YOU THINK IT MEANS: Products labeled this way aren't as likely to cause allergic reactions as other products.

THE REALITY: Cosmetics manufacturers aren't required to substantiate this claim, so it can mean whatever a company wants it to. "Some marketers use it in a meaningless fashion, while others test their products on panels of people with allergic potential," says Mort Westman, a cosmetic chemist and industry consultant in Oak Brook, Illinois.

WHEN IT'S DONE RIGHT: "No reputable company would ever release an allergenic product, which is why it's best to purchase brands that you know and trust," says Leslie Baumann, MD, a professor of dermatology at the University of Miami. Certain ones, such as Clinique and Dove, have built reputations on avoiding allergenic ingredients and testing for sensitivity. The claim is part of their heritage and is reflected in their marketing, says the CTFA's Dr. Bailey. Clinique, for example, uses the term allergy tested in its tagline, and every Clinique product is, in fact, tested multiple times on 600 people. If even one person has a reaction, the product isn't released.

Noncomedogenic

YOU THINK IT MEANS: It won't clog pores, which can lead to blackheads and whiteheads (comedones, in medical speak) and acne.

THE REALITY: The pore-plugging powers of ingredients are often evaluated by applying them to a rabbit's ear, which is a test that's far from foolproof, given that our skin is very different from rabbits' skin.

WHEN IT'S DONE RIGHT: Reputable companies always test final products—not just individual ingredients—for comedogenicity in controlled trials, says Ni'kita Wilson, a cosmetic chemist in Fairfield, New Jersey. A trained technician will examine panelists' skin and count their existing blemishes. After testers use the product as specified, their skin is reexamined. "If there's a dramatic increase in pimples, the company either won't release the product or won't make the noncomedogenic claim," says Wilson. Even with the claim, there's always a chance that a product will cause you to break out; if that happens, switch to another.

Oil Free

YOU THINK IT MEANS: There's no oil in the product to make your skin greasy or clog your pores.

THE REALITY: "Oil-free products don't contain ingredients—such as mineral oil or plant oils—classified by the CTFA as oils," says Wilson. But they might still include oil-like emollients, such as silicones, waxes, and vegetable fats, that can trigger outbreaks in susceptible people.

WHEN IT'S DONE RIGHT: It's virtually impossible to formulate cosmetics without oil-like ingredients. They're often used to give products a silky feel or to bind ingredients together. So if your skin is acne-prone, it's wiser to choose a noncomedogenic product over one labeled oil free.

CHAPTER 26

Take Off
10 YEARS!

Our experts help five women update their routines to achieve smoother, firmer, more radiant skin. Learn how you can see major results in minimal time

Who wouldn't want to turn back the hands of time to look 10 years younger. But it is possible to fade discoloration, stop sagging, banish breakouts, relieve redness, and fight the signs of aging. Here's how!

GOAL: FADE DISCOLORATION

DANA ENDICOTT, 41, UNION CITY, NEW JERSEY

Dana was concerned about discoloration around her cheeks and on her nose. These irregular patches of excess pigment, known as melasma, had progressively worsened over the last 2 years.

"Dana's going through an early menopause, so hormonal fluctuations are the likely cause," says Robin Ashinoff, MD, director of cosmetic dermatology at Hackensack University Medical Center in New Jersey. "Sun exposure worsens the condition, prompting cells to pump out more pigment, which is why it's most noticeable during the summer."

Old Routine

Dana's bare-bones approach—daily and nightly cleansing and moisturizing—allowed dead cells and clusters of melanin to build up and leave her complexion looking dull and uneven. Though she's careful to use a moisturizer with SPF 15 daily, it doesn't provide strong enough protection against UVA, the rays that trigger pigmentation.

New Routine

MORNING

Use a brightening face wash. A cleanser with lightening agents such as niacin (a B vitamin) helps inhibit the release of melanin, which is the pigment that colors skin.

Spot-treat with a bleacher. Applying a lightweight brightening serum with kojic acid, arbutin, or Sepiwhite to dark patches one morning a week fades splotches.

Apply SPF 30. Diligently wearing a moisturizer with a broad-spectrum sunscreen every day helps keep pigment from forming.

EVENING

Exfoliate while cleansing. Gently rubbing skin with a Buf-Puf or washcloth while using her face wash helps dissolve dead cells and fade mottling.

Target discoloration. A prescription bleaching cream such as Tri-Luma—which contains tretinoin (one of the age-reversing retinoids), hydroquinone to lighten, and cortisone to calm irritation—offers speedy results. Use according to your dermatologist's directions; otherwise you can exacerbate the very problem you're trying to treat.

Keep skin hydrated. A moisturizing cream packed with niacin improves tone and boosts radiance. Dr. Ashinoff suggests waiting at least 20 minutes before applying to avoid diluting the efficacy of the Rx lightener.

The Results

"Before my makeover, people assumed I was older than I am," Dana says. "Now that my spots have faded, people guess I'm in my early 30s. I sometimes have to show a picture of my 20-year-old daughter to prove I'm in my 40s!"

"I no longer look in the mirror and just focus on my spots. Now I see me."

Her essentials: AM/PM cleanser: NIA24 Gentle Cleansing Cream ($30; nia24.com); SPF: Aveeno Positively Radiant Daily Moisturizer SPF 30 ($14; drugstore.com); bleacher: Tri-Luma (from $175; by prescription); night cream: Burt's Bees Radiance Night Creme ($15; Whole Foods)

GOAL: STOP SAGGING

NANNETTE SMITH, 62, RICHMOND, VIRGINIA

Nannette started noticing changes in her skin about a decade ago, but she wasn't sure what anti-aging products worked best for her supersensitive complexion, which is also prone to hyperpigmentation.

"Darker skin doesn't wrinkle as much as Caucasian skin, but it does sag," says Pamela Royal, MD, a dermatologist in Richmond, Virginia. "But you have to be careful which products you choose, since even using a scrub that's too aggressive can cause discoloration."

Old Routine

Nannette had a decidedly hands-off approach to skin care: Other than occasionally washing her face, she didn't do much for fear of drying and irritating her delicate skin.

New Routine

MORNING

Choose a moisturizing cleanser. A mild face wash that's free of fragrance, colorants, and harsh detergents prevents dryness and inflammation that can often lead to unwanted pigmentation.

Protect skin by applying an antioxidant serum. Vitamins C and E and ferulic acid defend against free radicals that damage collagen, the proteins that keep skin from sagging.

Finish with a high-SPF sunscreen. Even darker skin can burn, so choose a broad-spectrum SPF 30 or above to ensure strong protection. Avoid sunscreens with titanium dioxide or zinc oxide, which can leave a white tinge on ethnic skin, suggests Dr. Royal.

EVENING

Prep skin for treatment products. Washing away dirt and grime with the same cleanser used in the morning allows anti-agers to seep in better.

Firm with Renova. To lower risk of irritation, use this collagen booster every third night, at least for the first 2 weeks. Apply every other day for the next 2 weeks, and build up to daily use. A little dab will do: Smear on a pea-size

WARMING TREND

Here are five products that heat up on contact to penetrate deep for potent anti-aging.

SHAVE WITH EASE: Aloe vera- and marshmallow extract-filled Bliss Thermal Shaving Cream ($18; drugstore.com) creates a friction-free glide for silky legs.

FIGHT FRIZZ: The volcanic ash in Pureology Thickening Masque ($36; amazon.com) plumps strands for added volume; UV filters keep color brilliant, longer.

BRIGHTEN UP: Exfoliating salicylic acid and vitamin A in Dermalogica AGE Smart MultiVitamin Thermafoliant ($48; dermalogica.com for locations) polish skin and soften wrinkles.

HEAL HEELS: With powerful pumice, Avon Foot Works Thermal Exfoliating Scrub ($8; avon.com) sloughs unsightly calluses and soothes tired feet.

DEEP CLEAN PORES: Gentle microbeads in Olay Warming Deep Purifying Cleanser ($9; drugstores) lift away dead cells, dirt, and makeup; green tea imparts a smooth finish.

For more self-heating lotions and potions, check out prevention.com/warmingbeauty.

amount 20 minutes after cleansing skin, avoiding sensitive areas such as your lips and upper eyelids.

Moisturize and minimize dark marks. Patting affected areas with a hydrating fade cream or serum made with the natural lighteners bearberry and soy helps even skin tone and restore your youthful glow.

The Results

"I was shocked at how quickly I saw changes, and I'm tickled to death about the wonderful improvement in my skin," Nannette says. "It's firmer and much more evenly toned. This routine has helped me finally take control of my appearance—talk about empowering!"

"I accept that aging happens, but I want to look my best. This routine has given me better skin than I thought possible."

Her essentials: AM/PM cleanser: Cetaphil Gentle Skin Cleanser ($8; drugstores); antioxidant serum: Aubrey Organics Sea Buckthorn with Ester-C Rejuvenating Antioxidant Serum ($16; Whole Foods); SPF: LaRoche Posay Anthelios SPF 40 Sunscreen ($30; CVS); retinoid: Renova (about $140; by prescription only); night cream: Dr. Susan Taylor's Rx for Brown Skin Advanced Botanical Brightener ($35; Sephora)

GOAL: BANISH BREAKOUTS
KATHY SLINSKY, 43, DARIEN, CONNECTICUT

Kathy can't remember a time when she didn't have a pimple or two (or three or four!). But her approach to battling blemishes was making her fine lines more noticeable.

"Skin becomes less oily with age, so acne products that worked in your 20s and 30s may become too drying," says Lisa Donofrio, MD, associate clinical professor of dermatology at Yale University School of Medicine.

Old Routine

Kathy attempted to dry out pimples by stripping her skin with aggressive cleaners and skipping moisturizer for fear of clogging her pores.

New Routine

MORNING

Wash with an antimicrobial cleanser. Products that contain triclosan or benzoyl peroxide kill acne-causing bacteria.

Layer on a lightweight lotion with SPF. An oil-free, noncomedogenic formula with built-in sunscreen keeps breakouts and skin aging at bay.

EVENING

Use an exfoliating cleanser. One with salicylic or glycolic acid clears pore-clogging cells.

Ramp up exfoliation. Avage, the most potent prescription retinoid, quickly heals acne as it fades discoloration and softens fine lines. To avoid initial irritation, apply a thin layer each night and wash off after 5 minutes.

Moisturize to soothe any side effects. Temper redness from the retinoid by hydrating with a night cream that contains anti-inflammatories such as feverfew and chamomile.

The Results

"Once I got on the right track, the changes came quickly: Within a week, my skin was blemish free. If only that had been the case during senior year!"

Her essentials: AM cleanser: PanOxyl Acne Facial Bar ($7.50; dermadoc tor.com); PM cleanser: Patricia Wexler, MD; Dermatology Acnescription Exfoliating Acne Cleanser ($16; bathandbodyworks.com); SPF: Cosmedicine Medi-Matte Oil Control Lotion SPF 20 ($45; Sephora); night cream: Aveeno Ultra Calming Night Cream ($14; drugstores)

GOAL: RELIEVE REDNESS

JEANNE MUCHNICK, 47, LARCHMONT, NEW YORK

A lifetime of unprotected sun exposure caught up with Jeanne 2 years ago, when red patches wouldn't go away.

"UV damages the collagen that keeps blood vessels small and invisible," says David Bank, MD, a dermatologist in Mt. Kisco, New York. Because they also impair skin's ability to stay hydrated, Jeanne battled dryness, too.

Old Routine

Jeanne cleansed day and night with aggressive exfoliators that exacerbated redness and dryness. Though she moisturized twice daily, her lotion was too lightweight, and she only used sunscreen sporadically.

New Routine

MORNING

Skip cleansing. Splashing with lukewarm water prevents dryness.

Layer on a serum packed with antioxidants. Ingredients such as vitamins C and E help neutralize free radicals, easing redness.

Apply an SPF 30. Vigilant use of a broad-spectrum sunscreen made with a potent UVA blocker such as avobenzone, Mexoryl, or Helioplex is a must for reducing ruddiness.

EVENING

Use a hydrating, nonfoaming cleanser. Wash with warm water and your fingertips; hotter temps and washcloths can inflame her skin type.

Renew with an Rx retinoid. Renova revs production of collagen, the fibers that strengthen capillaries and plump skin—making redness less noticeable.

Soothe with souped-up moisturizers. Creams with licorice root extract calm skin.

The Results

"After just 6 weeks, I could get away without a thick layer of foundation to camouflage my redness," Jeanne says.

Her essentials: AM cleanser: CeraVe Hydrating cleanser ($11.50; drugstores); antioxidant serum: Juice Organics Vitamin Antioxidant Serum ($20; drugstore.com); retinoid: Renova (about $140; by prescription only); night cream: Eucerin Redness Relief Soothing Night Creme ($15; drugstores)

GOAL: FIGHT THE FIRST SIGNS OF AGING
JAMEY DOBBS, 50, KNOXVILLE, TENNESSEE

Despite Jamey's hectic life with four kids and a busy new career, she is ready to get serious about skin care. Kimberly Grande, MD, a dermatologist in Knoxville, recommends a 24/7 approach, which means Jamey can't fall straight into bed anymore without even washing her face.

"Skin rejuvenates itself best at night, when it's not competing with sun exposure and other environmental assaults," says Dr. Grande.

Old Routine

Jamey's regimen was very haphazard: She cleansed and moisturized only every few days and relied on the sun protection built into her makeup. The result: "My fine lines were making friends. I would go to bed with one and wake up with three," she jokes.

New Routine

MORNING

Start with a mild cleanser. To avoid drying skin, lather only on the oilier T-zone (the forehead, nose, and chin).

Enlist anti-agers. A serum packed with peptides stimulates collagen production to smooth and firm skin.

Step up the sunscreen. After years of unprotected sun exposure while growing up in Texas, Jamey assumed the damage was done, but Dr. Grande assured her that it's never too late to start safeguarding skin. Studies show that regular use of sunscreen allows the skin to start repairing itself.

EVENING

Use the same face wash. The gentle fragrance-free formula removes dirt and makeup but keeps skin soft and supple.

Layer on a retinoid. To diminish fine lines and lighten sun spots, start with a product that contains a retinol or retinaldehyde, less irritating retinoids that are available OTC.

Quench with a potent moisturizer. A hydrating cream with a humectant such as hyaluronic acid or glycerin plumps wrinkles by drawing water to skin.

De-crinkle with an eye cream. Choose one made with peptides to fade lines by thickening this delicate tissue.

YOUTH BOOST IN A BOTTLE

Get a glow! This new slew of potions immediately gives skin a hint of tint and delivers long-term benefits.

THE PRODUCT: Olay Definity Color Recapture ($25; drugstores)

NOW: Optical diffusers (pigments that scatter light over the face) help skin look smooth and firm.

LATER: Niacinamide and glucosamine fade brown spots.

THE PRODUCT: Borba HD-Illuminating Light Effects Serum ($50; borba.com)

NOW: Microdiamonds reflect light for a soft, luminous complexion.

LATER: Kojic acid and vitamin C even tone and boost firmness.

THE PRODUCT: L'Oreal Paris Age Perfect Pro-Calcium Radiance Perfector Sheer Tint Moisturizer ($20; drugstores)

NOW: A subtle wash of color creates a fresh-faced appearance.

LATER: Beta hydroxy acid increases cell turnover to soften fine lines.

The Results

"I taped my routine on the bathroom mirror to help me stay on track, and it paid off," Jamey says. "Years of damage have been undone in just 3 months. I had no idea my skin tone could look this even. I thought that was what makeup was for!"

"Caring for my complexion didn't just improve my skin. It allowed me to pay more attention to myself."

Her essentials: AM/PM cleanser: Boots Expert Sensitive Gentle Cleansing Wash ($5; Target); serum: Olay Regenerist Daily Regenerating Serum ($18; drugstores); retinol: Eau Thermale Avene Retrinal 0.05% ($56; dermstore.com); eye cream: Derma E Peptides Plus Wrinkle Reverse Eye Creme ($27.50; dermae.com); night cream: L'Oreal Paris Skin Genesis Night Complex ($20; drugstores)

CHAPTER 27

BEAUTIFY Your Body

If signs of aging are breathing down your you-know-what, chin up, there's lots you can do

Time takes its toll not just on our faces but on every part of us. It leaves its biggest calling cards on our necks, hands, and feet. But you can fool even the savviest age guesser with the following new strategies.

FEEL GREAT ABOUT YOUR NECK

Tired of hiding your age underneath a turtleneck? Thank the hierarchy of skin care. Most of us have spent decades pampering our faces, only to have the wear and tear on our necks give us away. (Who knew the skin on your neck is the thinnest on the body, making it more susceptible to damage?) As it turns out, some of the very anti-aging products you use on your face can help your neck look younger, too. We've also uncovered the newest in-office treatments that, although expensive, are proven to give your face a prettier pedestal. Follow this guide and say good-bye turtlenecks, hello V-necks!

NECK NUISANCE: DARK SPLOTCHES

UV exposure overstimulates pigment-producing cells, causing blotchiness.

The fix: A bleaching cream that contains kojic acid or mushroom or licorice extract can lighten dark spots, but be patient: Results may take months. Use products made with hydroquinone cautiously; the fader can be irritating.

"This area is drier and more sensitive because it contains fewer lubricating oil glands," says Heidi Waldorf, MD, director of laser and cosmetic dermatology at Mount Sinai School of Medicine.

Anti-agers such as retinol or alpha hydroxy acid–based creams help to drive the lightening agents deeper into your skin, making them more effective. To reduce irritation, use them on your neck every third evening and slowly work up to nightly application.

A broad-spectrum sunscreen of at least SPF 15 worn daily can prevent more spots. For the best protection, look for one with avobenzone (aka Parsol 1789), Helioplex, or Mexoryl.

NECK NUISANCE: WRINKLES

Years of sunlight break down collagen fibers responsible for keeping skin youthful and firm.

The fix: Skin care products, including those containing retinol and peptides, can build collagen and smooth skin—even reducing the so-called tree-ring lines.

In-office options are considered the gold standard, says Ronald Moy, MD, a professor at the David Geffen School of Medicine at UCLA. One to consider: fractionated resurfacing, with lasers such as Fraxel and Affirm. They stimulate cell turnover and the production of fresh collagen by making thousands of microscopic wounds over 20 percent of your skin. Because the surrounding skin is left untouched, healing time is minimal. The slight redness it causes subsides within a few days. You'll see significant improvement: Fine lines are often reduced by up to 50 percent after five or six monthly treatments at $500 a pop.

NECK NUISANCE: TURKEY WATTLE

This fleshy flap of skin forms underneath your neck as a result of excess fat, loose skin, and weak muscles.

The fix: Liposuction performed under local anesthesia is a quick fix, says Yael Halaas, MD, a facial plastic surgeon in New York City. During the half-hour procedure, which costs around $2,500, small incisions are made behind the ears or below the chin; excess fat is vacuumed out via tiny suction tubes.

To reduce bruising and swelling, which can last up to 2 weeks, another option is ultrasound-assisted lipo, which employs sound waves that liquefy fat before it's suctioned out. (With either treatment, you'll need to wear a neck sling for 2 weeks to help skin re-drape properly.)

If you have excess skin, you might need to pair lipo with a neck lift to completely regain firmness. During the 1- to 2-hour procedure, which costs about $1,000 more, small incisions are made behind your ears or under your chin and then excess skin is trimmed, lifted, and sutured into place.

NECK PRODUCTS WE LOVE

SMOOTH SKIN: With light-reflecting technology, Benefit Firmology ($32; benefitcosmetics.com) restores a glow.

LIGHTEN SUN SPOTS. Mushroom extract in BeFine Food Skin Care Neck Cream ($24; CVS) evens out skin tone.

PREVENT DAMAGE. Daily use of L'Oréal Paris Collagen Remodeler Contouring Moisturizer for Face and Neck SPF 15 ($20; drugstores) fends off UV aging.

REDUCE SAGGING. The collagen boosters chlorella extract and hydroxyproline in Shiseido Benefiance Concentrated Neck Contour Treatment ($48; Macy's) tighten skin.

NECK NUISANCE: BANDING

These vertical cords appear when the platysma, the thin sheet of muscle that covers the neck, begins to stretch out of shape, says Dr. Halaas.

The fix: Botox injected directly into the platysma temporarily smooths the cords by relaxing the muscle. Each treatment costs about $500 and lasts approximately 4 months.

Surgery is a more permanent option. During a platysmaplasty, which runs about $4,000, the muscle is tightened and anchored through a small incision under the chin. Any post-op bruising and swelling should subside within a week. Then your age will be your secret to keep or reveal.

HELP FOR HANDS

Dry hands can be more than a nuisance; they can be painful as well. Here's how to get softer mitts in 5 minutes, help for when a moisturizer isn't enough.

The hot trend we've got our finger on? New at-home versions of spa treatments that incorporate heat to rejuvenate skin. "Raising the temperature of skin by a few degrees makes it more porous, so active ingredients are absorbed faster," says Donna Perillo, owner of Sweet Lily Natural Nail Spa in New York City. If the drying effects of indoor air have left your hands in need of more than a liberal dose of lotion, you're in luck. Here are three skin savers you're sure to warm up to.

Essence of Beauty Lotion Candle ($10; cvs.com): The vitamin E- and soy-based formula doubles as a leave-on paraffin treatment: Blow out the wick and immediately massage the warm liquid onto your skin.

76

THE PERCENTAGE OF WOMEN WHO STRUGGLE WITH DRY HANDS, ACCORDING TO NIVEA

Ulta Warming Hand Mask: ($14; ulta.com) This oil-rich mask self-heats as you rub it on; rinse off after 5 minutes.

Bath & Body Works Suddenly Sauna: ($15; bathandbodyworks.com) Pour water into the gloves, and they'll turn toasty in 2 minutes; slip them on after applying the moisturizer and wear for up to 20 minutes.

FOR FEET'S SAKE

A pretty nail polish goes a long way toward making feet look younger. But with each passing year, dryness, calluses, and discoloration seem to get a little worse. These simple solutions undo life's wear and tear to keep feet beautiful all year round.

FOOT PROBLEM: DRYNESS

Too few oil glands leave feet prone to dryness; with age, cell turnover slows, making the problem worse.

The fix: Hydrate daily. Restore softness by applying foot cream immediately after bathing, while skin is still wet.

"These formulas are heavier than body lotions so they seep into thicker skin," says Stuart Mogul, DPM, a podiatrist in New York City. For maximum benefits, look for one that also contains exfoliators such as lactic acid to improve penetration of hydrators like glycerin.

Get a prescription: If skin is extremely rough, see your dermatologist for an Rx lotion such as Keralac, which contains higher doses of healing ingredients.

Dry between toes after applying: Moisture collects there, encouraging bacterial growth.

FOOT PROBLEM: THICK TOENAILS

Unlike fingernails, which thin with age, toenails become harder and thicker due to constant pressure from shoes.

The fix: Coat nails nightly with Vaseline. "This makes them softer and easier to trim," says Mary P. Lupo, MD, a clinical professor of dermatology at Tulane University.

Clip and file correctly. To eliminate splits and the risk of ingrowns, trim nails into a square shape using a clipper. Aim to make them even with the tips of your toes, and smooth rough edges by filing lightly in long strokes using a fine-grade emery board.

FOOT PROBLEM: OVERGROWN CUTICLES

Excess skin builds up over time and attaches to the nail.

The fix: Soften cuticles every 2 weeks. Rub on cuticle oil and immerse feet in warm water for 10 minutes to loosen skin. Alternatively, apply a cuticle remover such as Dashing Diva Cuti-Peel ($7; dashingdiva.com); most contain allantoin, an ingredient that softens dead skin, making it easier to take off.

Push back and trim. Gently ease cuticles off the nail with an orangewood stick, and snip hangnails using a nipper.

FOOT PROBLEM: CALLUSES

These thick and hardened areas of skin form as a result of constant pressure and friction; genetics also plays a role.

The fix: Exfoliate daily. Use a foot file or pumice stone in the shower to buff away dead cells. "Water softens skin, making it easier to remove," explains Natasha Kurpas, a manicurist at the Rita Hazan Salon in New York City. Also, avoid overzealous sloughing (calluses protect feet, so don't file them down entirely) and razors, which can cut skin and lead to infection.

FOOT PROBLEM: YELLOWING NAILS

This discoloration is usually residual staining from red or darker polishes.

The fix: Buff superficial stains. Lightly filing nails erases surface marks.

FOOT CANDY!

SOFTEN SOLES. Peppermint- and cocoa butter-packed The Body Shop Peppermint Cooling Foot Lotion ($16; thebodyshop.com) refreshes, too.

GET RID OF CALLUSES. Easy-to-grip Microplane Foot Buffer ($20; microplane.com) reduces roughness. The orb catches dead skin.

WAKE UP TIRED FEET. When dissolved in cool water, Avon Watermelon Effervescent Foot Tablets ($5; avon.com) revitalize fatigued feet.

BLOCK BLISTERS. The aloe- and vitamin E-based Dr. Scholl's for Her Miracle Shield ($7; drugstores) dries to a powder finish that helps protect feet from rubbing that causes blisters.

FIGHT FLAKINESS. Exfoliating white sand in Olay Thermal Pedicure ($9; drugstores) smooths; the moisturizing formula heats up to relax feet.

HEAL HEELS. The intensely hydrating shea butter, coconut oil, and beeswax in Earth Therapeutics Cracked Heel Repair Push-Up Stick ($10; earththerapeutics.com) soothe painful dryness.

Bleach nails. Remove stubborn stains with weekly use of a nail brightener such as Barielle Nail Brightener ($16; barielle.com), which contains citric acid to fade discoloration. Or use the natural citric acid from a lemon, says Ji Baek, founder of Rescue Beauty Lounge in New York City and author of *Rescue Your Nails*.

Use a base coat. Applying this clear polish before painting nails creates a stain-fighting barrier.

Alternate shades. If you wear dark hues, go lighter every 3 weeks.

See your doctor. Persistent yellowing could be a sign of health problems.

SOUND ADVICE

TOP THREE WAYS TO SAVE YOUR SKIN

Here's skin-saving advice from *Prevention* advisor Mary P. Lupo, MD, clinical professor of dermatology at Tulane University School of Medicine and past president of the Women's Dermatological Society.

1. **DON'T SMOKE.** Smoking puts chemicals into your system that enhance free radical formation, explains Dr. Lupo. Free radicals cause your collagen to break down. Plus, smoking deprives all of your organs of oxygen, which is very important for the repair mechanisms of the skin, giving you a healthy glow. That's why smokers often have sallow complexions. To make matters worse, smoking decreases the oxygen content of your skin, so in an effort to get more oxygen, the capillaries dilate—and break. Those little broken capillaries on your face give an unhealthy appearance.

2. **DON'T GO TO TANNING BEDS.** The ultraviolet light in tanning beds is the longer wavelength of ultraviolet light that penetrates deeper into the skin and more actively destroys the collagen, says Dr. Lupo. Plus, the ultraviolet rays suppress your skin's immune system. They have a direct, detrimental effect on the T cells that help fight fungus, viruses, and skin cancer. So you're getting a dose of cancer-causing rays, *and* you're also suppressing your body's ability to counteract the damage. These detrimental effects of tanning beds are compounded when you also get natural sunlight. The two combined are worse than regular sunlight alone.

3. **START USING A RETINOID EVERY NIGHT WHEN YOU'RE IN YOUR TEENS.** Retinoids are the one thing that have been proven scientifically to reverse the effects of photoaging, says Dr. Lupo. You start photoaging in your teens—sometimes even earlier depending on where, and how, you live. Additionally, retinoids have been proven to build new collagen. And third, they help to prevent acne by preventing pores from getting clogged. The benefits of retinoids are cumulative, so the younger you are when you start using them, the better you'll look.

   It's best to get a retinoid prescription from a dermatologist, says Dr. Lupo. But the three over-the-counter preparations she suggests are Biomedic Retinol Cream, Help Me by Philosophy, and RoC Retinol.

PHOTO CREDITS

INDEX

Boldface page references indicate photographs. <u>Underscored</u> references indicate boxed text.